Healing with
Herbs A–Z

How to Heal Your Mind and Body with Herbs, Home Remedies, and Minerals

HANNA KROEGER

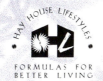

Hay House, Inc.
Carlsbad, CA

Published and distributed in the United States by:
Hay House, Inc., P.O. Box 5100, Carlsbad, CA 92018-5100
(800) 654-5126 • (800) 650-5115 (fax)

Edited by: Gretchen Lalik of Kroeger Herb Products, and Dee Bakker and Jill Kramer of Hay House
Designed by: Tom Morgan, Blue Design

Library of Congress Cataloging-in-Publication Data

Kroeger, Hanna.
  Healing with Herbs A—Z / Hanna Kroeger
   ISBN 1-56170-488-1 (hardcover)   p.   cm.
    1. Herbs—Therapeutic use. 2. Vitamin therapy. I. Title.
RM666.H33K764 1998
615'.321—dc21   97-51592
                                           CIP

ISBN 1-56170-488-1
First printing, June 1998
01 00 99 98 4 3 2 1
Printed in Hong Kong through Palace Press International

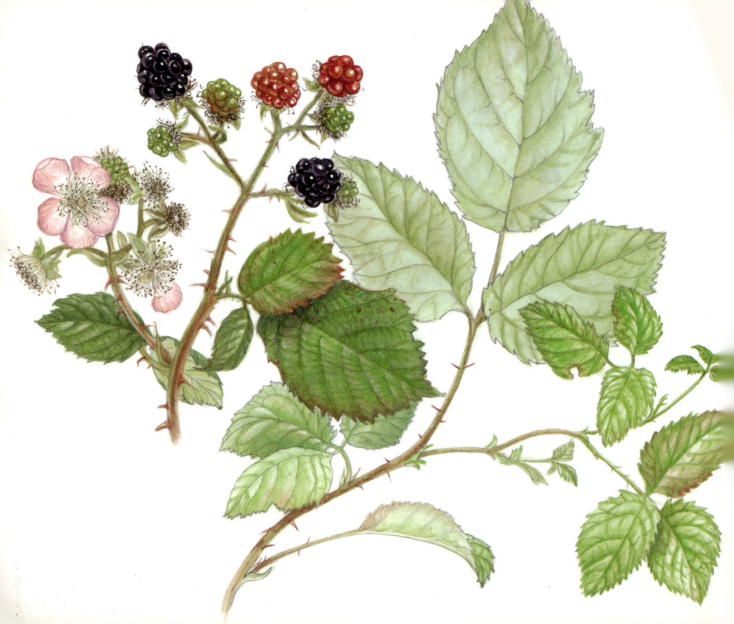

TABLE OF CONTENTS

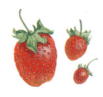

INTRODUCTION

Herbs heal the spiritual body. Herbs heal the aura. Herbs heal the subtle, vital energies of the physical body. Over the years, ever-increasing numbers of men and women have become involved with natural foods and herbs. In many hospitals, resorts, and sanatoriums in Europe, both herbs and foods, as well as medicine, are used in perfect harmony and to the good of humankind.

The following reference guide allows you to determine which herbs, home remedies, and minerals are right for you. Remember, in no way will good, natural, nonchemical or unadulterated food and a cup of good herbal tea interfere with your physician's work. Herbs do not interfere with your physician's prescriptions, but they go far beyond the healing of drugs by healing the spirit, by energizing the aura, and by strengthening the bio-life power. Your physician will be happy that you are more balanced—that you have more strength and endurance to ther illnesses.

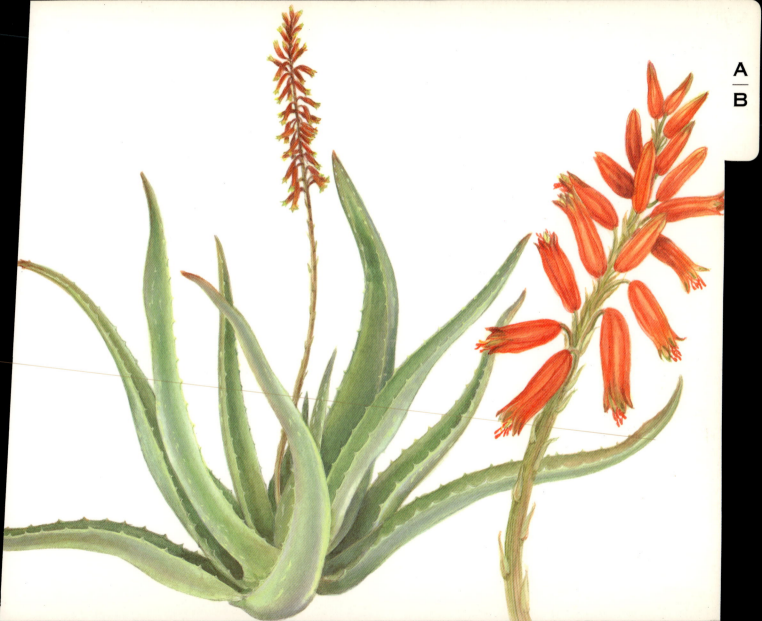

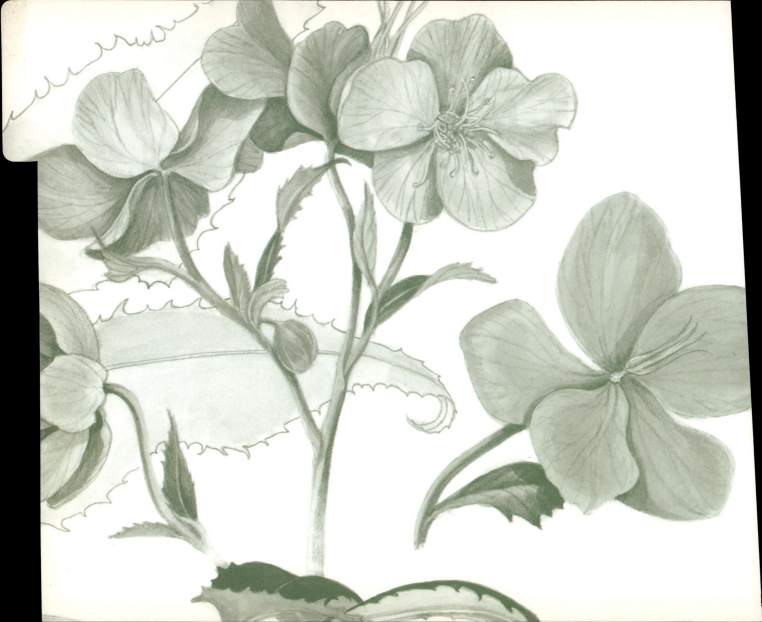

HERBS, HOME REMEDIES, AND MINERALS CHART

The following chart lists health concerns and the corresponding herbs, home remedies, and minerals that will help correct the problem. If not already in your kitchen, many of these homeopathic remedies, teas, and herbs can be found in your local health food store.

ABDOMINAL TENDERNESS

HOME REMEDIES
- Linden flower tea
- 12-herb tincture formula:* rub on navel

ACHILLES TENDON PAIN

HOME REMEDIES
- St. Ignatius's bean (*Ignatia amara*) (homeopathic)

ACID INDIGESTION

VITAMINS / MINERALS
- B1, B2, minerals from raw potatoes

HOME REMEDIES
- Yarrow tea: Drink 1/2 cup two times daily.

ACNE (SEE ALSO BOILS AND PIMPLES; PIMPLES)

VITAMINS / MINERALS
- A, C, B6 (young people)
- A, C, B2, E (common)

HOME REMEDIES
- For facial acne: Try homeopathic *Bellis perennris* (daisy).
- Dandelion, nettle, strawberry leaves: Single or together as tea.
- Charcoal tablets: Take two before each meal daily.

- Buttermilk and honey: Boil buttermilk; when thickened, add honey so it becomes a thick cream. Apply wherever needed.
- Walnut leaves
- Avoid all chocolate.

AGING: PREVENTING (SEE ALSO WEAKNESS)

HOME REMEDIES
- Lavender; Sage; Thyme
- Sarsaparilla root, dried: Bring 1 tsp. of sarsaparilla root and 1 cup of cold water to a boil and then turn down and simmer for 5 minutes. Drink 6 ozs. twice daily.
- Whey: Premature aging is a mineral deficiency. Whey has lots of minerals. It will keep muscles young, joints moveable, and ligaments elastic.
- 12-herb tincture formula*

AIDS, PREVENTION

HOME REMEDIES
- Take 1 tbl. lecithin granules and 1 egg yolk (fresh), mix thoroughly and add to juice (no citrus), water, or skim milk. Do this twice a week. This will liquefy the virus so it cannot attach.

For more information, see page iii.

ALCOHOL (DRINKING TOO MUCH)

VITAMINS / MINERALS

- B1: 100 mg. three times daily

HOME REMEDIES

- Cucumber (enzyme called erepsin): Reduces the alcohol's intoxicating effect
- Honey: Removes alcohol from the blood extra fast

ALCOHOLISM (CANDIDA ENCASED IN LIVER)

VITAMINS / MINERALS

- Alcoholics suffer from severe vitamin C, B, and zinc deficiencies.
- B-complex, B1, B12, E, choline, inositol, pantothenic acid, niacin

HOME REMEDIES

- Sometimes there are parasites in the pancreas; take a specific remedy to help.
- Chromium and vanadium mixed together: Take 1 tsp. twice daily to reduce the desire for alcohol.
- Take 1 tbl. Epsom salts in the morning and 1 at night.
- The herb ginkgo biloba is a help for alcohol cravings.
- Thyme tea: Helps stop the desire

ALLERGIES (GENERAL)

VITAMINS / MINERALS

- A, G, B6, B12, E, pantothenic acid, L-histidine

HOME REMEDIES

- Wild plum bark syrup
- Sage: Use on a piece of buttered whole-grain bread (rye or wheat).
- Orange rind or peelings mixed in a tea: Relieve stuffed up nose and clogged air passages and healthful sleep results.
- Banana: For energy and nerves; hinders allergies
- Honey: To relieve symptoms, you should use honey from your own neighborhood. It can act as an antihistamine.
- To cleanse lymphatic system: Every hour drink 4 oz. pure water. Do this for 2 days. Then make a vegetable broth and drink on the hour 6 oz. broth, and on the hour 4 oz. water.
- All allergies have two factors in common: chemical poison and parasites. See a physician to find your parasites.

ANEMIA (SEE ALSO SPLEEN)

VITAMINS / MINERALS

- A, B2, B6, B12, copper, iron

HOME REMEDIES

- Manukka raisins, molasses: Contain extra minerals
- Beet juice and yellow dock contain iron.

- Eggplant: Reduces enlarged spleen and increases red blood corpuscles and hemoglobin
- Grape juice, blackstrap molasses: 2 tsps. molasses in 1 glass grape juice
- Grape juice: 1 glass juice and 1 egg yolk
- Lentils contain protein supplies and iron of the best quality.
- Pumpkin seeds: Chew well.
- Raisins and ½ grapefruit: 2 ozs. dark raisins 3 times daily for 1 day; ½ grapefruit twice daily second day; alternate for 3 weeks.
- Spinach: Blood builder; raw is best.
- Wine: ½ glass red wine, ½ glass water, 2 egg yolks

ANGINA PECTORIS

HOME REMEDIES
- Apple cider vinegar: Heat apple cider vinegar. Wet a Turkish towel with warm vinegar. Apply to the back and chest of angina sufferer until help arrives.

ANKLES, PAIN

HOME REMEDIES
- St. John's wort (*Hypericum perforatum*) (homeopathic)

ANKLES AND FEET (PAIN)

HOME REMEDIES
- Pokeroot tea: Drink 2 cups daily and soak feet.

ANKLES, PAIN IN JOINTS

HOME REMEDIES
- Potato peelings: Simmer one handful in 2 cups of water for 15 minutes. Strain and take 2 tbls. in 1 glass of water 4 times daily for 14 days. After several days, legs and ankles should be more normal size.

ANKLES, WEAK

HOME REMEDIES
- Scotch pine tea: Make a strong tea and wrap compresses around ankles.

ANOREXIA NERVOSA (REFUSAL TO EAT, CAUSING SEVERE WEIGHT LOSS)

VITAMINS / MINERALS
- Possible zinc deficiency
HOME REMEDIES
- Good sources of zinc: lean meat, poultry, fish, shellfish, oatmeal, whole wheat bread, peas, lima beans, egg yolks, brewer's yeast, wheat germ, milk,

and yogurt
- Cloves help to stimulate the appetite, making it easier to recover.
- Rub your earlobes several times a day.

ANUS, BITING

HOME REMEDIES·
- Peony *(Paeonia officinalis)* tea

ANUS, BURNING

HOME REMEDIES
- Blue flag *(Iris versicolor)* tea

ANUS, ITCHING (SEE ALSO LIVER)

HOME REMEDIES
- Ground ivy tea: 1 cup a day

ANUS, PAINFUL

Home Remedies
- Ginger tea: $1/2$ cup three times a day

ANXIETY

VITAMINS / MINERALS
- Lack of chromium and magnesium
HOME REMEDIES
- Borage and thyme tea

APATHY

HOME REMEDIES
- Saw Palmetto *(Sabal serrulata)* (homeopathic)

APPETITE, LOSS OF

VITAMINS / MINERALS
- B6, B12
HOME REMEDIES
- Apples help regain appetite.
- Alfalfa in small amounts creates sound appetite and improves digestion.
- Caraway and eggplant improve appetite.
- Homeopathic: Dandelion *(Taraxacum officinale)*

APPETITE, LOSS OF IN CHILDREN

HOME REMEDIES
- Cranberry juice or sauce

ARCHES, FALLEN

HOME REMEDIES
- Comfrey root tincture: Apply overnight on soles of feet.

ARM-SHOULDER SYNDROME (PAIN)

VITAMINS / MINERALS
- B-complex, B12, folic acid

ARMS (PAIN IN UPPER LEFT)

HOME REMEDIES

- Watch the heart. Sometimes the muscles in the arms hurt because of arsenic poisoning in the muscles.

ARTERIES

HOME REMEDIES

- Yogurt and applesauce: 1 dish daily to keep arteries clean.
- Aloe vera aids in assimilation, circulation, and elimination.

ARTERIOSCLEROSIS (HARDENING OF ARTERIES)

VITAMINS / MINERALS

- A, B12, E

HOME REMEDIES

- Apple tree bark tea
- Parsley: Keeps arteries clear
- Combine: Brussels sprouts, alfalfa, garlic, vitamin F, whey, violet, hyssop, clover; eat 4 cups per day.
- Distilled water, lecithin
- Indian remedy: Tea of sassafras. Also 1/2 tsp. cream of tartar, twice weekly.

ARTHRITIS

VITAMINS / MINERALS

- A, B-complex, B1, B15, D, E

HOME REMEDIES

- Trace minerals from alfalfa seeds
- When diet is too alkaline: Add calcium, protein from pumpkin seeds, and take okra tablets for extra minerals.
- Apple cider vinegar, honey, water: Combine 2 tsps. each vinegar and honey in 8 ozs. of water. Take 3 times daily with meals.
- Avocado seed: Pound, make strong tea, and apply to skin.
- Celery, parsley, and celeriac: Eat celery and parsley every day or juice them and eat celeriac.
- Five foods: Black cherry juice; peanut oil, 2 tbls.; alfalfa seeds, juice, or tablets; celeriac or celery root; liquid rice B-complex.
- Flaxseed: Can be used externally or internally
- Garlic: Crush, spread in cloth like butter on bread. Wrap poultice around arthritic joint 2 to 12 hours, which will raise a large blister full of water. This will break and run out, drawing the disease out of the joint. Heal the burn with aloe vera juice and see amazing results.
- Lemon, orange, grapefruit: Grate 1 lemon, 1 orange, 1 grapefruit. Add 2 tsps. cream of tartar, 2 tbls. Epsom salts, 1 quart water. Drink 2 ozs. 3 times daily.

- Oil of wintergreen: Rub on joints; also kerosene on joints.
- Eat strawberries, cranberries, asparagus, and Swiss chard.
- Whey: Mix 2 tbls. with 1 tbl. lecithin and 8 tbls. of vegetable broth. Take 3 times daily for several months.
- Brown paper: Make layers, sew between two layers of flannel, and use as a bed covering. The DMSO pine residue relieves pain and heals.
- Willow bark: Make tea.

ARTHRITIS, DEFORMATION OF HANDS AND FEET

HOME REMEDIES

- Comfrey root: Make and apply warm compresses.
- Cabbage leaf: Heat and apply overnight.

ARTHRITIS, PRONE TO

HOME REMEDIES

- Phosphorus

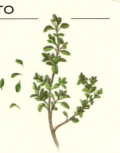

ASTHMA

VITAMINS / MINERALS

- A, C, B-complex, choline, inositol, lecithin, E

HOME REMEDIES

- Anise tea
- Cinnamon; Wild cherry bark
- Elecampane and quebracho: Gallbladder flush
- Thyme powder mixed with honey. Dosage: 1 tsp. every hour.
- Wild plum bark: Make syrup and take 1 tbl. 4 times daily. Make a pillow and sleep with it. Good for hay fever, too.
- Wormwood: Boil in apple juice.
- Lemon juice: Take 2 tbls. before each meal.
- Radish and honey: Grate black radish; add honey. Before going to bed take 1 tsp. of the mixture.
- Go on a ½ day fast. The time you don't eat, take 2 quarts of water, soak green pineapples in it, and let sit for 2 hours. Drink from that fluid for the other half of the day (all you want). Do this for 10 to 14 days.
- Red onion, (raw), juice mixed with raw sugar. Dosage: 1 tsp. every hour.
- Sunflower seeds: 1 quart sunflower seeds in ½ gallon water; boil down to 1 quart of water. Strain, add 1 pint honey; boil down to a syrup. Give 1 tsp. 3 times daily.
- Homeopathic remedy for adults: yerba santa (*Eriodictyon glutinosum*).

ASTHMA ATTACK

HOME REMEDIES
- Cranberry juice concentrate: One tsp. can stop an attack. To make your own: Boil 1 pint water and 1 pound cranberries until done, then refrigerate. Dosage: 1 tsp.
- Put hands in hot water.

ASTHMA, IN CHILDREN

HOME REMEDIES
- *Thuja occidentalis* (homeopathic)

ASTIGMATISM (MYOPIC) (SEE ALSO MYOPIC ASTIGMATISM)

HOME REMEDIES
- Tiger lily (*Lilium tigrinum*) (homeopathic)

ATHLETE'S FOOT

VITAMINS / MINERALS
- A

HOME REMEDIES
- Bathe feet in rosehips tea or lemon juice or follow suggestions on Clorox bottle.
- Spinach seed and onion seed: Simmer 2 tbls. of the seeds in 1 quart of water for $1/2$ hour; then soak feet in the water.
- Quaw bark tincture: Apply externally.

ATTENTION DEFICIT DISORDER (ADD)

VITAMINS / MINERALS
- B1 supplement will help.

HOME REMEDIES
- Birthright Tea heals the trauma. *Plumbum metallicum* clears the lead poisoning (a possible cause of ADD).

AUTISM

VITAMINS / MINERALS
- Calcium, magnesium, vitamin B6, and chromium for the hypoglycemia

HOME REMEDIES
- A specific remedy for parasites in the pancreas
- Avoid sugar and food allergens.

BACKACHE, AFFECTING HIPS AND SACRUM (WALKING STOOPED)

HOME REMEDIES
- Horse chestnut

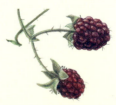

BACKACHE, IN CHILDREN

HOME REMEDIES

- Alfalfa seed, dill seed

BACKACHE, LUMBAR REGION

HOME REMEDIES

- Pokeroot tea: Simmer root; 2 cups daily.

BACTERIAL INFECTION

HOME REMEDIES

- Cabbage: It's anti-inflammatory, antibacterial, and encourages new cell growth. Onions: Absorb bacteria; can be used to help disinfect sickroom.
- Goldenseal root (*Hydrastis canadensis*) (homeopathic)
- Black pepper: Kills bacteria and can be used as a food preservative
- Garlic; cinnamon; fiber in whole-grain foods

BAD BREATH

VITAMINS / MINERALS

- Possible zinc deficiency

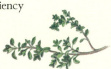

HOME REMEDIES

- Sometimes a disturbed function of the gallbladder or liver or both. May also be a sign of major gum disease.
- Try sipping thyme tea or chewing on dill seeds to freshen breath.
- Caraway seed and anise seed, mixed together
- Homeopathic: *Arsenicum album; Baptisia tinctoria*

BALDNESS

VITAMINS / MINERALS

- PABA, biotin, folic acid, inositol

BEDSORES

VITAMINS / MINERALS

- C, E, copper

BED-WETTING

VITAMINS / MINERALS

- B1, B-complex, E, magnesium

HOME REMEDIES

- Avoid sugar, simple sugars, and allergenic foods.
- Bistort tea, equisetum tea, violet leaf tea: Serve no later than 4 hours before bedtime.

- Cinnamon: Helps prevent bed-wetting and also promotes sleep.
- Cuttlefish *(Sepia); Calcerea phosphorica*

BEE STING (IN THE MOUTH OR THROAT: THIS IS A SERIOUS ACCIDENT)

HOME REMEDIES

- Salt: Take 1 tsp. of salt and put in the mouth at once. It has prevented many from strangling to death.
- Onion: Rub raw onion on the area.

BELCHING

HOME REMEDIES

- Papaya tablets have an enzyme that will prevent belching.
- Saw palmetto tea
- Try massaging earlobes.
- Avoid carbonated beverages, eat slowly, avoid chewing gum, and avoid foods with high air content.
- Artichoke: Brings a clear urine and increases the flow of bile. It is also claimed that it keeps the arteries smooth and a person free from weak digestion. Useful for albumin in the urine and jaundice.
- Soup: Small bowl at the beginning of meal is stimulating to the bile.

BIRTHMARKS

HOME REMEDIES

- Castor oil: Apply for several months.

BITES (SEE ALSO INSECT BITES; MOSQUITO BITES)

HOME REMEDIES

- Dog or cat bite: Assess damage to determine if you need medical attention.
  Then thoroughly wash the wound with soap and water. Continue washing for 5 full minutes. Do not shy away from a tetanus shot. Take Homeopathic Thuja afterwards.
- Rattlesnake bite: Wet some salt and wrap the bitten arm or leg in a salt pack, making sure the bite gets an extra dose of salt. Then, RUSH to your physician.
- Poisonous spider: Consult physician. Use the homeopathic Glondirine as well.

BLACKHEADS

VITAMINS / MINERALS

- A

HOME REMEDIES

- Cucumber: Cut a piece and rub over face. Also, cover face with cucumber peelings, the cut side to the skin.
- Strawberries: Rub fresh berries over face.

- Wash face with hot water, and then sprinkle with cold water.
- Use soap and water, lathering freely; dry, rinse thoroughly. Afterwards, sponge with witch hazel. Repeat daily.

BLADDER

VITAMINS / MINERALS

- A, B6, Magnesium

BLADDER, HEMORRHAGE

HOME REMEDIES

- Peach tree bark tea: Drink 3 cups daily.
- Comfrey root: Drink 3 cups daily.

BLADDER, INFECTION

VITAMINS / MINERALS

- A, B6, C, E

HOME REMEDIES

- Trace minerals from uva ursi
- Collinsonia root tea
- Cranberry juice (drink plenty)
- Pomegranate: Juice it and mix 1/2 cup with 1/2 cup water, and sip it. It is even better as a fruit eaten twice a day.
- Take a wool blanket and spread on your bed. Place a cotton sheet over it, and sleep on it. (Will also help with kidney problems.)

BLADDER, PAIN

HOME REMEDIES

- Marshmallow root: If due to a cold, take 1 tbl. marshmallow root in 1 cup water. Drink hot.
- Pomegranate: As a juice, 1/2 cup with 1/2 cup water. Better as fruit; eat one twice a day.

BLADDER, STONES

HOME REMEDIES

- Carrot leaves, parsley tea: 1 quart a day for 3 days; then just 2 cups a day for 2 weeks.

BLADDER, WEAK

HOME REMEDIES

- Pumpkin seed: Take 1 tsp. three times daily or more if desired.
- Chickpea

BLEEDING, CUTS

HOME REMEDIES

- Cover the cut with unglazed brown paper moistened with vinegar.

BLEEDING, FEMALE (SEE ALSO FEMALE BLEEDING)

HOME REMEDIES

- Okra

BLEEDING, GUMS (SEE ALSO GUMS)

VITAMINS / MINERALS

- C, E, P, K2, chromium

HOME REMEDIES

- Black pepper: Freshly ground, it's loaded with chromium, which is needed for proper functioning of the pancreas and heart.
- Lemons: Wash and cut 6 lemons in little pieces. Cover with 1-1/2 quarts of water and bring to a boil. Turn off heat and let sit for 25 minutes. Strain and set aside until cool. Take 6 ozs. 2 times daily for 10 days. In case of bleeding gums, hold juice in your mouth, also.
- Papaya seeds: Chew 1 tsp. papaya seeds 4 times daily and spit out after chewing thoroughly.

BLEEDING, INTESTINAL

HOME REMEDIES

- Shepherd's purse tea: Drink 1 cup twice a day.

BLEEDING, TOOTH (AFTER EXTRACTION)

HOME REMEDIES

- Black tea: Moisten one tea bag with warm water and apply to tooth.

BLISTERS

HOME REMEDIES

- Homeopathic: Buttercup (*Ranunculus bulbosus*) for blisters in the palm of your hand.
- Sage: Eat or make tea and drink for blisters in the mouth.
- Arnica and violet tea: Hold in mouth and drink (for blisters in the mouth).

BLOATEDNESS

HOME REMEDIES

- Caraway and fennel: Take equal parts, grind seeds in blender.
- Sage with peppermint: Make tea.
- Fennel: 1 tsp. fennel. Bring to a boil in 8 ozs. of water. Simmer 10 minutes. Strain 1 to 2 cups for adults; children 1/2 cup.
- Anise: Make a very diluted tea and give a few drops as needed.
- Gentian tea: Use 1/2 to 1 cup a day.

BLOOD, BUILDERS

VITAMINS / MINERALS

- B6

HOME REMEDIES

- Egg yolk: Mix with some concord grape juice. Terrific blood builder.
- Apricots: Eat two dried, twice daily, or soak and blend them.
- Blackstrap molasses: 2 to 4 tsps. daily.
- Beet and grape juice: 1 part red beet juice, 2 parts dark grape juice. Take 2 tbls. 3 times daily.
- Carrots, watermelon seed, bananas: All blood builders
- Red clover tea

BLOOD, CLEANSER

HOME REMEDIES

- Lemon juice, honey, and water: Take 6 ozs. every 2 hours.
- Take 1 tsp. sanicle to 1 cup of boiling water.
- Take 5 parts red clover and 1 part chaparral: Make tea and drink 2 cups daily.
- Take 1 tsp. sassafras tea to a cup of boiling water (strong cleanser).
- Take 1 tsp. sheep sorrel to 1 cup of boiling water (strong cleanser).

BLOOD, POISONING

HOME REMEDIES

- Cranberries: Boil 1 quart cranberry juice with 8 cloves and 1 tsp. cinnamon. Add 1 quart of water and drink this in a day.

BLOOD PRESSURE

VITAMINS / MINERALS

- B-12, B-complex, lecithin, garlic: for elasticity of the vessels.

HOME REMEDIES

- Parsley: Make parsley tea and also add parsley to salads and soups.
- Parsley, celery, garlic: Eat plenty of parsley and add garlic and celery. Or buy a juicer, juice the vegetables, and drink 6 ozs., twice daily.
- Apples: Eat two a day.
- Turnip tops: Boil turnips tops as you would spinach. Eaten with rice once every day lowers blood pressure.
- Watermelon seeds: Dilate the blood vessels, lower pressure, and improve kidney function.
- Homeopathic: Wild indigo (*Baptisia tinctoria*), Hawthorn (*Crataegus oxycantha*), Cone flower (*Echinacea angustifolia*)

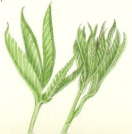

BLOOD PRESSURE, HIGH

VITAMINS / MINERALS

- B1, B-complex, lecithin, garlic for elasticity of vessels, potassium

HOME REMEDIES

- Oranges and lemons: 3 oranges, 2 lemons. Cut into pieces. Boil in 1 quart of water for 15 minutes. Then add 2 tbls. of honey. Boil another 10 minutes. Strain and drink 6 ozs., 3 times daily, before meals (not for diabetics).
- Mistletoe and angelica: Combine 2 tsp. of each in 1 quart water; bring to a boil and drink 2 to 3 cups a day.
- Garlic regulates blood pressure.
- Peas and beans (for potassium)
- Homeopathic: *Uranium nitricum*

BLOOD PRESSURE, LOW

VITAMINS / MINERALS

- B1, B6, B-complex
- Copper, iron, niacin

HOME REMEDIES

- Cayenne: Add to your food.
- Apricots: Mix with dark raisins. Eat 2 tbls., three times daily.
- Protein
- Homeopathic: *Cactus grandiflorus*

BODY ODOR

VITAMINS / MINERALS

- Zinc, calcium/magnesium, plant-derived colloidal minerals

HOME REMEDIES

- Chlorophyll: Everything green has chlorophyll. Take plenty of green drinks or buy liquid chlorophyll to combat body odor. Parsley contains chlorophyll.
- Drink tomato juice daily.
- Lots of green, leafy vegetables; alfalfa

BOILS

VITAMINS / MINERALS

- A, C, bioflavonoids, E

HOME REMEDIES

- Onions: Put onion poultice over a boil to bring it to a head.
- Tomato: Cut the stem out of a ripe tomato; turn tomato over the boil to bring it to a head. (Indian remedy)
- Garden sage and cornmeal as a poultice
- Flaxseed poultice
- See your physician.

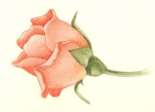

BOILS AND PIMPLES

HOME REMEDIES

- Nutmeg: Combine $^1/_3$ tsp. nutmeg (freshly ground), 1 tsp. honey, and 4 to 5 ozs. hot water. Drink three mornings in a row. Don't drink it for three days. Repeat nine times.

BONES, BRITTLE

VITAMINS / MINERALS

- B-complex, B12, C, E
- Calcium (bonemeal), potassium

HOME REMEDIES

- Cabbage builds bones.
- Bananas (potassium) keep bones healthy.

BONES, BROKEN

HOME REMEDIES

- Comfrey root
- Wild geranium tea
- Take an orange towel and sleep on it. Also, do it when bones are healed and still give trouble.

BONES, PAIN

HOME REMEDIES

- Comfrey root tea
- Comfrey root tincture

BONES, TENDON AND MUSCLE INJURIES

HOME REMEDIES

- Comfrey root compresses
- Arnica root is best.

BONES, WEAK

HOME REMEDIES

- Fenugreek seed: Take in tablet or capsule form.

BOTULISM

HOME REMEDIES

- Apple cider vinegar: 2 tsps. in 7 ozs. of warm water and sip slowly. For children, add honey.

BOWELS

HOME REMEDIES

- Alfalfa helps them move.
- Black pepper tea will help running bowels.
- Barley is excellent food for children suffering from inflammation of the bowels.

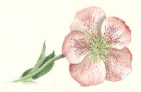

BOWELS, BLEEDING

HOME REMEDIES

- Cinnamon bark tea: ¹/₂ cup 4 times a day will heal all bleeding bowels. Or chew on cinnamon bark until you can visit your physician.

BOWELS, CLEANSING

HOME REMEDIES

- Flaxseed: Gently simmer for about ¹/₂ hour, then let stand where it will remain hot for 1 or 2 hours longer. Combine 2 tbls. in 2 cups of boiling water; let it boil down to 1 cup. Add sugar to taste. Add the juice of lemon if you want. Drink the whole cupful at bedtime and swallow all the seeds. Take about once a week, every 4 days, or more often if needed. It is harmless.
- Molasses and lemon: When there is lots of gas present, combine 1 tbl. molasses, the juice of 1 lemon, and 1 quart of hot water.
- Always check for protozoa and worms.

BOWELS, DROPPED

HOME REMEDIES

- Prickly pear

BRAIN, FOOD

VITAMINS / MINERALS

- B12, folic acid, gotu kola to strengthen concentration.

HOME REMEDIES

- Combine 1 lb. sunflower seeds, ¹/₄ lb. almonds, 1 lb. wheat; grind up and eat 2 heaping tbls. a day.
- Cardamom is an eye and brain food.
- Brain cocktail: Combine 1 cup barley, 1 cup coconut juice, 1 tbl. lecithin. Honey, if desired
- Coconut: Eat the meat and drink the milk.
- Leeks: Cut, boil, and use in soups or salads.
- Dried apple peelings made into tea are full of silicon, which will strengthen the brain.
- Almonds; Almond oil: Only 1 tsp. daily will improve memory.
- Oats help memory.
- Cloves in tea will heighten memory.
- Sage: On slice of lightly buttered rye bread
- Eyebright in capsules or tablets strengthen memory.
- Take 2 mustard seeds to improve memory.
- Take hawthorn tablets or as tea to combat mental dullness.
- Lemon balm to promote youth and strengthen the brain
- Take Dulcamara or purple cone flower to clear up mental confusion.
- Basil: Eat it or wash your hands, arms, and face with basil tea.

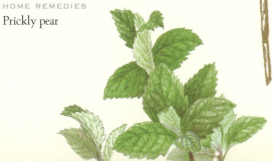

- Homeopathic: Honey bee (*Apis mellifica*)

BRAIN, TUMOR

HOME REMEDIES

- Tofu: Shave head, apply tofu over head, and change the compress when tofu gets yellow.
- Tomato: Use raw crushed tomato in a cheesecloth poultice.

BREAST, LUMPS OR PAIN

HOME REMEDIES

- Bag balm available at veterinary supply house

BREATH, BAD (SEE BAD BREATH)

BREATH, SHORTNESS OF

HOME REMEDIES

- Black tea: A cup of black tea often relieves breathing difficulty until you find a doctor's help.
- Red onion juice: Bring to a boil, add honey, simmer for 15 minutes. Take 1 tsp. every hour. One tbl. raw onion juice with 1 tsp. sugar.

BRIGHT'S DISEASE (KIDNEY TROUBLE) (SEE ALSO KIDNEY INFLAMMATION)

HOME REMEDIES

- Watermelon seed: For 2 days eat nothing but watermelon. Eat always by itself.

BRONCHITIS

HOME REMEDIES

- Flaxseed: To 1 pint of flaxseed tea, add the juice of 2 lemons, and 3 tbls. honey. Take 1 tsp. every half hour until relieved.
- Myrtle leaves: Contain Myrtal, an active antiseptic. Use as a tea.
- White hellebore: For elderly with bronchitis
- Myrrh: Use in chest rubs for congestion.
- Helpful herbs: Daffodil, lungwort, plantain, or 12-herb tincture formula*
- Take Echinacea, either as tea or in capsule form.

BRONCHITIS, PRONE TO

VITAMINS / MINERALS

- Phosphorus

BRUISES

VITAMINS / MINERALS

- C, bioflavonoids, pantothenic acid, K2, rutin

* *For more information, see page iii.*

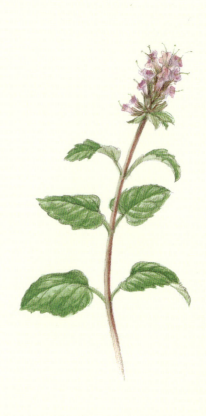

HOME REMEDIES

- Chestnut leaves or alfalfa provide K2.
- Crushed peach leaves applied as a poultice
- Solomon's seal or daisy tea poultices
- Apply a hot milk and crushed seed (fenugreek) poultice.

Burns

VITAMINS / MINERALS

- C, E

HOME REMEDIES

- Aloe vera: Apply to burns.
- Cold water: Place under cold water until all pain is gone. (For minor burns; if serious, begin cold water treatment and call for medical help at once.)
- Some dip a burn in cold fresh cream if available.
- Black tea
- Egg white: Slightly beaten and applied to first- and second-degree burns will take away pain.

Bursitis

HOME REMEDIES

- Take 2 parts magnesium and 1 part calcium.
- Homeopathic: *Arsenicum metallicum*
- See a chiropractor.

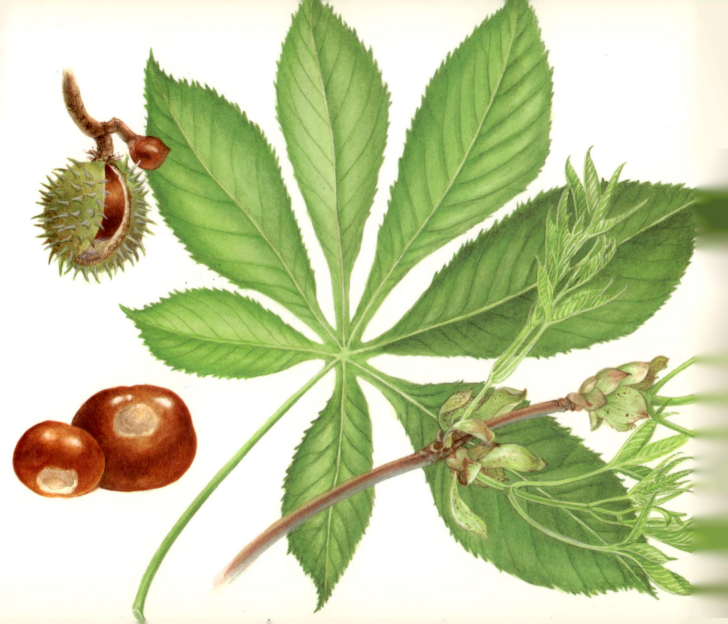

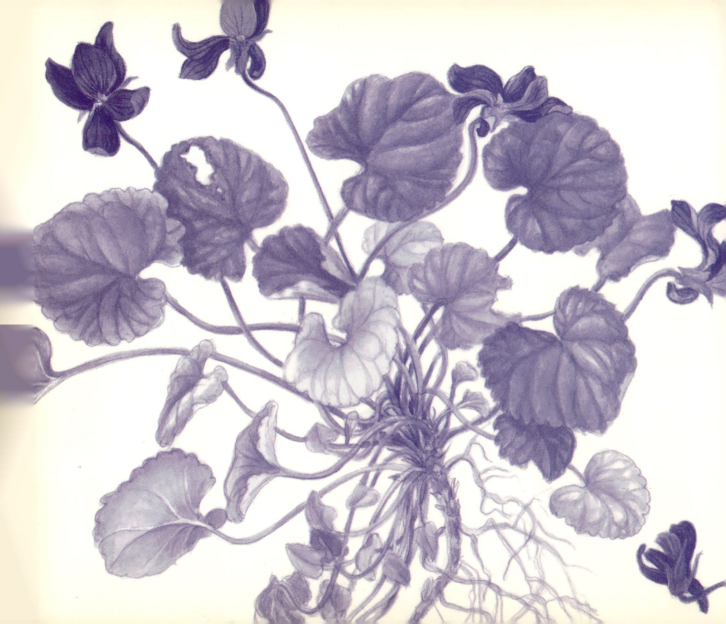

CALCIUM (NEED MORE)

HOME REMEDIES

- Broccoli contains more available calcium than milk or other sources.
- Cauliflower: A very good calcium supplier

CALLUSES AND CORNS

VITAMINS / MINERALS

- A, C

HOME REMEDIES

- Lemon and castor oil
- Take a piece of lemon and tie over corns overnight. Repeat with new lemon every night.
- Rub peppermint oil on calluses.
- Soak feet in very warm water for 5 minutes. Then buff with pumice to remove dead skin.
- Homeopathic: Buttercup (*Ranunculus bulbosus*) (for corns)

CANCER

HOME REMEDIES

- Concord grape juice: Every morning for 6 weeks, drink 1 quart of juice from the time you wake up until noon, with no other food. After noon, eat normally. Emphasize almonds, asparagus, and other fruits and vegetables, with no heavy protein after 2 P.M. Used in Europe with outstanding results.

- Orange peelings: Dried, boiled; use for cancer patients having pain, particularly if cancer is in mouth or tongue.
- Cabbage: Valuable for its healing properties

CANCER (PREVENTION)

VITAMINS / MINERALS

- Iodine (from asparagus) may be helpful in preventing cancer and other cell-destroying diseases.

HOME REMEDIES

- Garlic: Found to block the formation of colon cancer and may prevent other types
- Cabbage: Contains ingredients that prevent cancer. Important dietary addition.
- Asparagus: Contains substances that assist body in normal cell formation
- Antioxidants protecting against cancer: apricots, cantaloupe, carrots, citrus fruits, kale, parsley, spinach, sweet potatoes, turnip greens, winter squash, yams.
- Broccoli, cucumber, eggplant, pepper, and tomatoes: Contain plant steroids that block estrogen promotion in breast cancer
- Tomatoes and red grapefruit: Contain "lycopines," active chemical ingredients that protect against cancer
- Green tea, berries: Contain catechins that protect against cancer

CANDIDA ALBICANS (IRRITABLE BOWEL SYNDROME)

HOME REMEDIES

- Borage and thyme
- Rosemary: Thought to encourage the immune system
- Savory: Antibacterial, antifungal, and antiviral

CANKER SORES

VITAMINS / MINERALS

- B6, niacin, B2

HOME REMEDIES

- Sage: Use sage tea for mouth sores (or sore eyes). Or apply one inch of powdered sage against the sore.
- Apply goldenseal or raw onion to sore.

CARPAL TUNNEL SYNDROME

VITAMINS / MINERALS

- B12, B6, calcium, magnesium, zinc

CATARACTS

VITAMINS / MINERALS

- A, B2, B-complex, C, E, trace minerals from angelica root

HOME REMEDIES

- Combine equal parts yellow onion juice with honey. Mix well; use 1 or 2 drops in eyes twice daily.
- Coconut: Take the fresh juice from a coconut and with an eye dropper apply as much as the eye can hold, then apply hot wet cloths over the eye. Remain lying down and keep the towels hot for 10 minutes.
- Horseradish: Good for cataracts and inflammation of the eyes. Grate the root and eat raw or make broth.
- Natural cheddar cheese, sage honey: Eat 2 ozs. of cheddar cheese twice daily, put 1 drop of sage honey in each eye.
- Bean pods: 2 ozs. in 1 1/2 quarts water. Boil for 20 minutes and drink 6 ozs. 3 times daily.

CATARRH

HOME REMEDIES

- Horseradish: 1 tsp. several times a day

CATARRHAL DEAFNESS

HOME REMEDIES

- Garlic

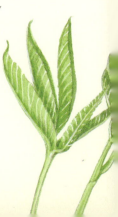

CELLULITE

HOME REMEDIES

- Eggplant: Slice and place in slightly salted water for about 20 minutes or more to remove the bitterness. Eggplant skin is extremely helpful. Peel the eggplant ½ -inch thick. Boil the peelings until done. Season with kelp or dulse. An excellent antidote to tumors and cellulite.
- Sage: Add to bathwater. (May also use sage oil.)

CHOLESTEROL

VITAMINS / MINERALS

- C, bioflavonoids, B-complex, E, F, choline, inositol, magnesium, lecithin

HOME REMEDIES

- Cranberries: 2 tbls. cranberry sauce once daily or 1 cup of juice a day
- Alfalfa sprouts: Use to dissolve cholesterol deposits.
- Apple: 1 a day
- Garlic, onions, leeks, and chives inhibit cholesterol synthesis and protect against carcinogens.
- Cayenne: When taken in capsules may reduce buildup

CHOREA

VITAMINS / MINERALS

- A, B1, B6, magnesium

CIRCULATION

VITAMINS / MINERALS

- Vitamin E deficiency

HOME REMEDIES

- Cardiac cocktail: 1 tbl. paprika, 1 tbl. vinegar. Gradually substitute cayenne in place of paprika as soon as you can tolerate it. For serious cases, take 1 cup of this in warm water twice daily.
- Tansy: Aids circulation to the uterus
- Fennel, ginger: Circulatory stimulants
- Rosemary, lily of the valley (Convallaria majalis) (homeopathic), and ginseng help circulation.

CLOTS

VITAMINS / MINERALS

- C, E, bioflavonoids, rutin, and minerals from white oak bark tea

HOME REMEDIES

- White oak bark tea

COLDS

VITAMINS / MINERALS

- A, C, iodine, calcium, trace minerals from elderflower and peppermint

HOME REMEDIES

- Celery: Increases the appetite; good in curing mucous conditions
- Combine: Cloves, cinnamon, sage, and bay leaves; boil in apple juice.
- Kale: Aids resistance to colds; has natural sulfur and lots of vitamins.
- Lemon balm, garlic, or cayenne pepper: Deter colds, flu if taken at the onset
- White and red onions: Make a soup from raw onions, season with Tamari or other broth and eat.
- Broccoli: Its natural sulfur strengthens resistance to colds.
- Thyme: For resistance to colds or prevention of colds, take thyme tea (1 cup a day).
- Grapefruit: Grate the skin of a grapefruit very fine. Add the juice of 1/2 grapefruit and fill cup with hot water. Grapefruit contains a substance similar to quinine.
- Indian remedy: For chest cold, mix turpentine and coconut butter to a paste, rub on hot wool cloth, and apply to chest or back.

COLD SORES

HOME REMEDIES

- Carrots: Take two, finely grated, place between 2 layers of cotton cloth and apply to sores. Change every 2 hours.
- Brewer's yeast, milk, meat, or soybeans: Sources of lysine, which helps block reproduction of herpes virus.
- Tea bags: Apply wet, black tea bags to canker sores.
- Use olive leaf compound.

COLIC

HOME REMEDIES

- Fennel: Add 1 tsp. seeds to 1 cup water. Bring to boil, then simmer for about 10 minutes. Strain, and give children only 1 tsp. in water.
- Gentian: Make tea, and give 1 tsp. in cup of warm water to children.
- Caraway and anise: Combine and make tea.
- Yam: Soothing properties help colic.
- Allspice; cinnamon: Both relieve colic.
- Dill tea: Diluted.
- Fenugreek tea: Drink.

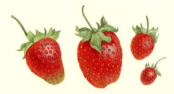

COLITIS

VITAMINS / MINERALS

- A, C, B-complex from rice polishing, E, F, magnesium, potassium from bran, trace minerals from white oak bark and goldenseal root
- Take calcium for a spastic colon.

HOME REMEDIES

- Comfrey tea, Fenugreek tea, wild blackberry or red oak bark tea, creamed papaya, charcoal, bananas relieve colitis.
- Flaxseed tea: Soak flaxseed in plenty of water overnight, then bring to a boil and simmer for 5 minutes. Drink 3 to 4 times a day.
- Carrots: Boil until done, then blend or mash them, and eat. Also drink 6 to 7 ozs. of carrot juice twice daily.

COLON, INFLAMMATION AND IRRITATION

VITAMINS / MINERALS

- Calcium: Try extra calcium when the abdomen is distended and bloated.
- Take B1 to strengthen.

HOME REMEDIES

- Irish potato peel and flaxseed meal: Boil a handful of potato peelings in plenty of water. Add 1 tbl. of flaxseed meal to 1 quart of potato peel water and drink 1 cup warm during the day until 1 quart is gone. Do this for 10 to 14 days.

- Rutabaga is excellent for a weak colon. It is food for the friendly bacteria in the colon and strengthens the membranes of the colon. Boil potatoes with rutabagas, mash them, and eat with butter and salt.
- Nutmeg: Combine 1/2 tsp. in hot water for distended abdomen (without nausea).
- Linden flower tea or 12-herb tincture formula*: For abdominal tenderness.
- Pears, rhubarb: Colon cleansers

COMPLEXION, CLEARED

HOME REMEDIES

- Cucumber juice with water. Or place slices of cucumber over face where needed.

COMPLEXION, GENERAL

HOME REMEDIES

- Drink 16 ozs. prune juice and 1 gallon apple juice each day for 3 days.

CONGESTION

HOME REMEDIES

- Foot bath with mustard draws blood out of head. For lungs, a mustard plaster with whole wheat flour; also excellent for kidneys.

* For more information, see page iii.

CONJUNCTIVITIS

VITAMINS / MINERALS

- B2

HOME REMEDIES

- Place raw potatoes on eyes (grated or sliced).

CONSTIPATION

VITAMINS / MINERALS

- B, C, sodium, trace minerals

HOME REMEDIES

- Figs and prunes: Soak 1 fig and 3 to 5 prunes in warm water overnight. Next morning, drink the juice and eat the fruit.
- Pears: 2 raw pears at bedtime. No water with them.
- Flaxseed: Soak 1 tbl. flaxseed with 1 tbl. raisins (currants are best) in 1 cup water. Next morning, eat them before breakfast. Or mix and soak flaxseed with prune juice. Take 1 or 2 tbls. daily.
- Squash with caraway and cream
- Raw apple: At bedtime chew an apple very carefully and drink a glass of water with it.
- Oranges, thyme: Good digestive tonics

CORNS AND CALLUSES

VITAMINS / MINERALS

- A

CORNS ON FEET, SENSITIVE

HOME REMEDIES

- Buttercup
- White cabbage: Grate cabbage, add hot water so it is comfortable to your feet. Soak them for 10 to 20 minutes.
- Lemon: Soak your feet in warm water for about 15 minutes, then cut a small piece of lemon peel and place the inside of it against the corn, tying it on, and let it stay there all night. Do this for 3 nights, and the corn should lift off.
- Epsom salts: Add to warm water; soak feet.
- Massage feet, and never wear tight shoes.

COUGH, DRY

HOME REMEDIES

- Potato peelings: Boil, sweeten with honey. Take 1 tbl. several times a day.
- Onion: Boil cut onions in apple cider vinegar. Add honey. Take 1 tsp. every hour.

COUGH, PHLEGM

HOME REMEDIES

- Ginger tea several times: 6 ozs.

COUGH, IN CHILDREN (CRAMPING)

HOME REMEDIES
- Boil bread in milk. Make a poultice over throat.

COUGH SYRUP

HOME REMEDIES
- Mix 4 drops eucalyptus oil in 1 cup of honey. Take 1 tsp. as needed.
- Dates, figs, sage: Combine 1 lb. dates, 1 lb. figs, 1 oz. sage, and 4 quarts distilled water. Boil all ingredients for 1/2 hour, strain, and boil this syrup down to 1 quart. Take as needed.
- Onion syrup: Take a yellow onion and make a hole in it. Fill hole with honey or raw sugar. Set it in a saucer and after an hour brown tasty syrup drops out. Excellent for children and adults
- Honey: Mix 1/2 honey and 1/2 lemon juice.

COUGH, WHOOPING

HOME REMEDIES
- Wild cherry bark: 1 tsp. 3 times daily
- Sage: Add 1 tbl. to 1 pint water; take 1 tsp. 5 times daily
- *Drosera rotundifolia*: Homeopathic remedy

CRAMPS, IN LEGS

VITAMINS / MINERALS
- Calcium lactate, B1

CRAMPS, MENSTRUAL

VITAMINS / MINERALS
- Calcium lactate, B1

CRAMPS, IN SOLES AND PALMS

HOME REMEDIES
- Ginger tea

CROHN'S DISEASE

VITAMINS / MINERALS
- Eat foods rich in vitamin E.

HOME REMEDIES
- Protozoa Kit
- Olive leaves: Counteract both protozoa and viral infections.

CUTS

HOME REMEDIES
- Cloves: Anesthetic properties relieve pain.
- Apple juice and olive oil: Mix and use as an antiseptic.

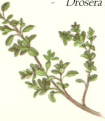

CYST FORMATION

VITAMINS / MINERALS

- Calcium

HOME REMEDIES

- Trailing arbutus (*Epigaea repens*): Homeopathic remedy

DANDRUFF (SEE ALSO HAIR)

VITAMINS / MINERALS

- E
- Lack of vitamin B can result in dandruff.

HOME REMEDIES

- White beets: Cut beets and boil in water until water is almost gone. Strain and take this water to moisten the scalp for 2 to 3 weeks.
- Coconut oil: Secure a small amount of pure coconut oil; rub in your hair for a few days and dandruff should disappear.
- Willow leaves: Boil a handful of leaves. Strain and wash your hair and scalp in it. Put a little concoction aside and dampen the scalp a little every day. (I found this recipe in an old herb book. I was amazed at the result.)

DEAFNESS

VITAMINS / MINERALS

- A, B12, E, F, iodine, niacin

DEODORIZER

VITAMINS / MINERALS

- Zinc

HOME REMEDIES

- Chlorophyll: Everything that is green has chlorophyll. Take plenty of green drinks or buy liquid chlorophyll to combat body odor.
- Eat some parsley after onions or garlic.

DEPRESSION

HOME REMEDIES

- Take extra pantothenic acid and vitamin B6.

HOME REMEDIES

- Two-thirds of all mental cases are kidney cases. Drink juice of 1 pomegranate in the morning, 1 persimmon at noon, and 1 wineglass full of grapefruit juice in the evening; keeps you in good humor.
- Black snakeroot: Indians chewed this root to calm the nerves and to alleviate depression.
- Lemon balm and daisy tea: A calming effect
- Borage tea: Helpful for grief, anxiety, and depression
- Anise and thyme teas
- Oranges, oats, and rosemary are helpful.
- Garlic: Burn the garlic skin slowly on an incense burner to help right away; it's a mild tranquilizer.

- Clove concentrate: Bruise a handful of cloves, steep in boiling water, then simmer for a few minutes. Do not reduce water too much or it will be too strong. Take 1 tsp. added to 1 cup of hot water. Or try clove tea.

DERMATITIS

HOME REMEDIES
- Oatmeal bath

DIABETES

VITAMINS / MINERALS
- (See your physician before treating yourself for diabetes.)
- B1, B2, B6, B12, niacin, C, E, lecithin, potassium, chromium, inositol, magnesium, zinc, acidophilus

HOME REMEDIES
- Avocado: Combine avocado with agar-agar (dry), lime juice, and raw rolled oats. Drink plenty of distilled water between meals.
- Blackberry leaf tea, blueberry leaf tea, or oat straw tea: Boil and drink 4 cups daily.
- Devil's claw: capsules
- Dwarf leaf tea: Drink 2 cups a day.
- Garlic: Helps regulate blood sugar levels; known to be beneficial in adult onset diabetes
- Paprika (zinc) will save eyesight in diabetics.
- Take 2 raw string beans daily.

- Jerusalem artichoke and parsley leaves are good.
- Watercress: Make a big salad out of one bunch of watercress for lunch.
- White figs: Make compresses over throat.

DIAPER RASH

VITAMINS / MINERALS
- A, D
- Vitamin A and D ointment is the best remedy. Be sure to dry diapers in the sunlight after washing.

DIARRHEA, CHRONIC

VITAMINS / MINERALS
- B6, C, F, calcium, magnesium

HOME REMEDIES
- Apples: Raw and finely grated will stop diarrhea in children.
- Arrowroot starch: Take 1 tsp. arrowroot. Make a paste with water and stir into 7 ozs. boiling water; add applesauce to taste.
- Blackberries: As a juice or as wine; or drink dried blackberry root tea.
- Black tea: 1 or 2 cups without sugar, sipped slowly
- Black pepper: Use as a tea for running bowels.
- Iceberg lettuce has a natural opium that is quite constipating.

- Oak bark tea; rice gruel; ripe, raw grated apples; slippery elm; strained carrots; cinnamon; cardamom; rice gruel; nutmeg: All relieve diarrhea.

DIGESTION

VITAMINS / MINERALS

- A, B, C, and E

HOME REMEDIES

- Alfalfa seed: Improves digestion. Use it as a tea after meals. Add 1 tsp. alfalfa seed to 1 cup cold water, bring to a boil, then turn the heat off. Let sit for 3 to 5 minutes.
- Flaxseed: It's soothing to an irritated digestive tract. It coats, heals, and nourishes. Take 2 tbls. of flaxseed to 1 quart of water. Simmer for 20 minutes, strain, and drink 1 cup of the warm mixture every 2 hours. For best results, alternate with carrot juice: 1 hour carrot juice, the next hour, flaxseed tea.
- Sage tea: Aids in protein digestion. Drink 1 cup 2 times daily.
- Basil, celery: Aid in digestion of protein, increase appetite, and are good for mucous.
- Zucchini: Wash zucchini and cut into pieces. Steam or boil with a little water; place on plate and sprinkle with ground almonds. Good for weak digestion.

- Fruit skin: Peel pears, apples, pineapples, peaches, apricots (or whatever you have).
  Take the peelings and simmer 3 to 5 minutes in plenty of water. Drink 7 ozs. several times a day for digestive problems.
- Garlic, nutmeg, cardamom, lettuce, spinach, oranges, ginger, thyme, papaya are digestive aids.

DIGESTION, IN CHILDREN

HOME REMEDIES

- Apple concentrate: Take 2 tsps. of concentrate in water before meals.

DISC TROUBLE

VITAMINS / MINERALS

- E, B-complex, C, pantothenic acid, B12, sulfur

DIURETICS

HOME REMEDIES

- Cucumber: A good diuretic, containing a hormone needed by the pancreas to produce insulin. It is also for skin troubles.
- Seeds: Take equal parts of caraway, fennel, and anise; 1 tsp. each for 1 cup of water.
- Parsley root tea

DIURETICS, FOR KIDNEY STONES

HOME REMEDIES

- Use cucumber juice or tea from avocado leaf. Or take 3 tsps. of brown cord seed and put in 1 pint of water. Allow to steep, then drink 1 cup daily. This is also said to be good for gallstones.

DIVERTICULITIS

VITAMINS / MINERALS

- B-complex from rice bran, E, folic acid, F, iron, sulfur, magnesium

HOME REMEDIES

- Eat no wheat; drink fennel tea to relieve bloatedness.

DIZZINESS

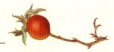

VITAMINS / MINERALS

- B1, B12, C, niacin, calcium, iron

HOME REMEDIES

- Rinse mouth with 1 tbl. of apple cider vinegar.

DIZZINESS, WITH DEAFNESS

HOME REMEDIES

- Take 1 tsp. horseradish every morning.

DOUCHE, HYGIENE

HOME REMEDIES

- Combine 1 pint apple brandy, 1 tsp. sea salt. Shake. Use 2 tbls. to 1 quart water. Excellent.

DROPSY

VITAMINS / MINERALS

- Potassium, C, E

HOME REMEDIES

- Broom tops: Take in capsules or as tea.
- Potato peelings: Boil peelings and drink 6 ozs. twice daily.
- Elder flowers: 2 cups daily.
- Horseradish in apple juice: Take 1/2 cup 3 times a day.
- Combine: 1/2 gallon apple cider; 1 handful parsley, crushed; 1 handful horseradish, crushed; 1 tbl. juniper berries. Put in cider, let stand 24 hours in a warm place before use. Take 1/2 glass 3 times a day before meals.

DRUG ADDICTION

HOME REMEDIES

- Epsom salts: Place 3 to 5 pounds of Epsom salts in a tub of hot water; let person soak for 20 minutes.

- From Denmark: Boil equal parts of carrots, onions, potatoes, celeriac (celery root). Take once a day for 7 days. Add salt and butter.

DRUG RESIDUE

VITAMINS / MINERALS
- Chromium and vanadium

HOME REMEDIES
- Lima beans: Make a healthful dish of lima beans, bell peppers, and sweet potatoes. Eat this once a day for 7 days.
- Chaparral tea: Two cups a day (or capsules) for heroin deposits.
- Tobacco leaf tea: Add to bathwater.
- Oats and celery root (celeriac): Eat to combat morphine habit.

DUODENAL ULCER

HOME REMEDIES
- Calamus root: Let sit in cold water overnight. Warm it in the morning (do not boil). Drink $\frac{1}{2}$ cup 4 to 5 times daily.
- Comfrey root tea: 2 cups daily
- 12-herb tincture formula*

For more information, see page iii.

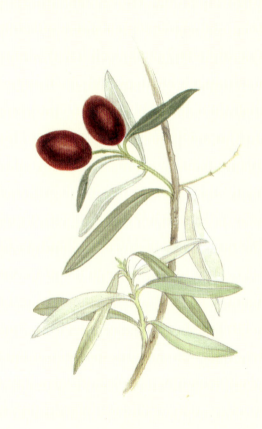

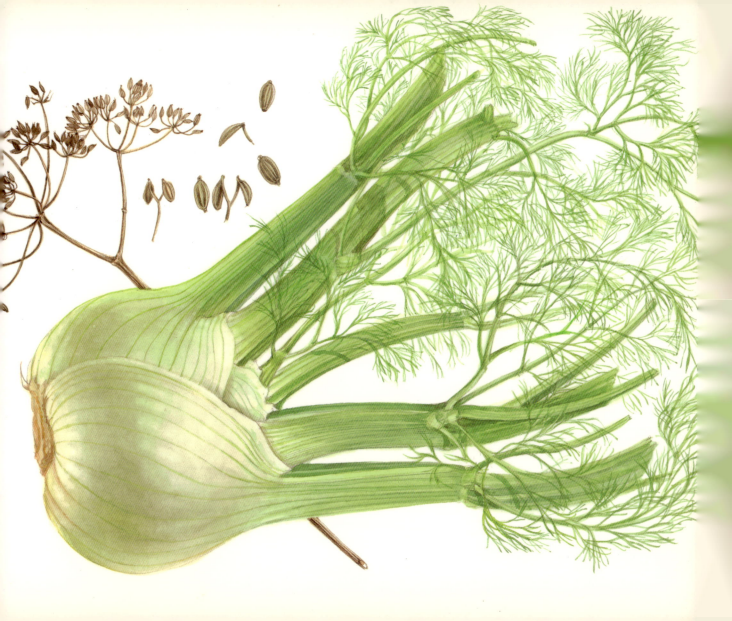

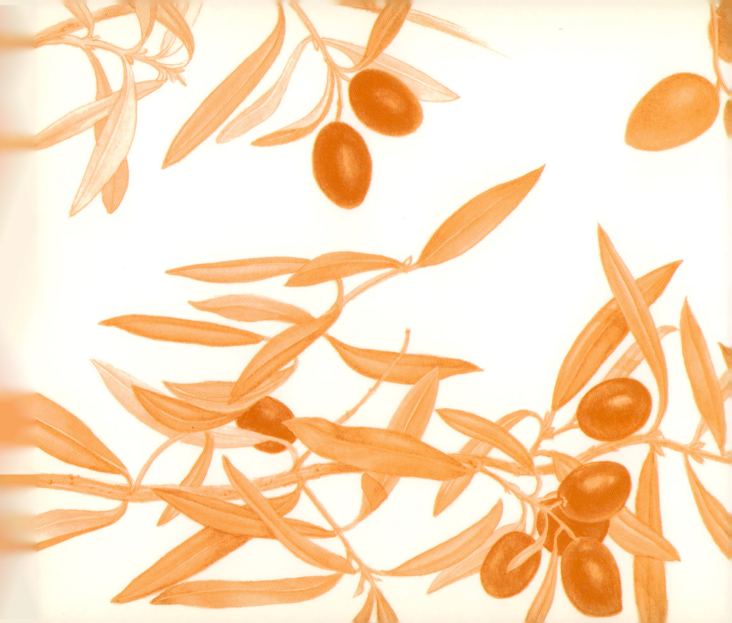

ECZEMA, SCALP

HOME REMEDIES
- Pansy (*Viola tricolor*) tea

EMOTIONAL SENSITIVITY

HOME REMEDIES
- Thuja tea (*Thuja occidentalis*)
(homeopathic)

EMPHYSEMA

VITAMINS / MINERALS
- A, B-complex, C, E, folic acid, friendly bacteria, aloe vera juice for trace minerals

ENDOMETRIOSIS (TUMORS ALL THROUGH THE UTERINE WALL)

VITAMINS / MINERALS
- B, C, inositol

HOME REMEDIES
- Dr. Carlton Fredericks says, "Absolutely no carbohydrates—not even bananas." Take 1,000 mg. choline and 500 mg. inositol with each meal. Stress B with C, 6 a day. Douche with alum root for bleeding. In 10 days, pain will leave. Keep up for 6 weeks.

ENERGY

VITAMINS / MINERALS
- B1, B-complex, lecithin, pantothenic acid, iron

HOME REMEDIES
- Grapes supply a lot of energy.
- Blackstrap molasses provides minerals and iron.
- Flaxseed: Let 1/2 tbl. flaxseed steep in 1/2 pint hot water; drink twice daily.

EPILEPSY

HOME REMEDIES
- Mistletoe (*Viscum album*) (homeopathic)

EPILEPTIC TYPE OF CONVULSIVE DISORDER

VITAMINS / MINERALS
- B6, calcium, magnesium

EXHAUSTION, NERVOUS

VITAMINS / MINERALS
- B-complex, B12, C, E, F, pantothenic acid

HOME REMEDIES
- Silicon herbs
- Whey powder: Take 1 tbl. twice daily.
- Thyme tea: Drink.

EYELIDS, CHRONIC INFECTION

VITAMINS / MINERALS
- A, B-complex, C, calcium

EYELIDS, SWOLLEN

HOME REMEDIES
- Primrose: Place well-beaten egg whites over closed eyes.

EYES, ACHING

VITAMINS / MINERALS
- Calcium fluoride

EYES, BURNING

VITAMINS / MINERALS
- A, B2, Eyebright herb for trace minerals
HOME REMEDIES
- Eyebright tea: Drink 2 cups daily.

EYES, CATARACT (SEE ALSO CATARACT)

HOME REMEDIES
- Bean pods: 2 oz. bean pods in 1 1/2 quarts water, boil for 20 minutes, and drink 6 oz. 3 times daily.

EYES, CONJUNCTIVITIS

HOME REMEDIES
- Raw potato: Place on eye.

EYES, AND DIGESTION

HOME REMEDIES
- Bell pepper (increases pepsin)

EYES, FARSIGHTED

HOME REMEDIES
- Lack of protein: You need more.

EYES, HEMORRHAGE

HOME REMEDIES
- Linden flower tea: Drink cool, 2 cups daily.

EYES, INFLAMED

HOME REMEDIES
- Castor oil: Apply to eyes.
- Elder flower tea: Apply externally and drink as well.
- Eyebright tea
- Red potato slices: Apply to eye.
- White lily leaves: Apply to eye.

EYES, LOSS OF VISION FROM DIABETES

VITAMINS / MINERALS
- Zinc

HOME REMEDIES
- Paprika (Hungarian is best)

EYES, LOSS OF VISION FROM TOBACCO

VITAMINS / MINERALS
- B12, folic acid

EYES, MUSCULAR WEAKNESS

HOME REMEDIES
- Linden flower tea: Drink cool, 2 cups daily.

EYES, PAIN

HOME REMEDIES
- Raw potato: Poultice over eye

EYES, PINKEYE

HOME REMEDIES
- Potatoes: Raw, grated potatoes over the closed eye. You may also take thin slices of raw potato and cover eye. It will release pain and the redness will go away. Red potatoes are best.

EYES, PROBLEMS WITH

HOME REMEDIES
- Cardamom: Eye and brain food
- Raw red potatoes: Grate 1 raw potato and use as a poultice over the eyes for 1 hour every day. Will improve eye conditions. Even cataracts have been known to be greatly benefited.

EYES, RETINAL BLEEDING

VITAMINS / MINERALS
- C, B1, bioflavonoids, rutin

HOME REMEDIES
- Raw potato compresses
- Paprika (Hungarian): 1 tsp. on your food 3 times daily.

EYES, STIES

HOME REMEDIES
- Eyebright (*Euphrasia officinalis*) (homeopathic)
- Castor oil
- Burdock root tea: Drink it and apply it.
- Black tea: Make a poultice, place moist over the eye, and bandage it overnight.

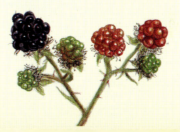

EYES, TIRED

VITAMINS / MINERALS

- A, B2, C, E, Eyebright for trace minerals

HOME REMEDIES

- Pure maple syrup: Take 1/2 to 1 tsp.
- Dr. Hohensee promoted the following formula: Juices of 1/2 potato, 1/2 onion, and 1/4 green pepper. Drink 8 ozs. of this 1/2 hour before supper. Eyes get clearer after 30 days.
- Red potatoes: Apply raw poultices.

EYES, TRAUMA (HARD BLOW)

HOME REMEDIES

- Comfrey root compresses

EYES, WATERING (EXCESSIVE)

HOME REMEDIES

- Euphrasia and Eyebright: Homeopathic

EYES, WEAK

HOME REMEDIES

- Rue tea: Drink 2 cups daily.

FACIAL MUSCLE, PAIN

VITAMINS / MINERALS

- B12, folic acid

FACIAL NEURALGIA

HOME REMEDIES

- Raw plantain juice: Apply over painful area.

FAINTING

VITAMINS / MINERALS

- E, B-complex, B6, manganese

HOME REMEDIES

- Lavender tea

FAT DEPOSITS

HOME REMEDIES

- Carrot juice: Through vitamin and mineral content, it helps the body release energy from the fat stores. It does not store well and should be made up fresh and drunk immediately if possible.

FATIGUE, CHRONIC

VITAMINS / MINERALS

- A, B-complex, B12, C, E, pantothenic acid, niacin, folic acid, trace mineral

FEAR

VITAMINS / MINERALS

- Niacin, B-complex, C, magnesium

HOME REMEDIES
- Rosemary tea, cinnamon tea, lavender tea: Equal parts

FEET, ACHING

VITAMINS / MINERALS
- Benzene

HOME REMEDIES
- Hot pepper: If hot peppers upset your stomach, sprinkle hot peppers on the soles of your feet and put on your socks. Hot peppers and radishes contain benzene, which is needed for proper functioning of feet and sinuses.

FEET, BURNING

VITAMINS / MINERALS
- Niacin, B-complex, C, magnesium

HOME REMEDIES
- Tomato: Try tomato slices on the soles of your feet.

FEET, CRAMPS

VITAMINS / MINERALS
- Sulfur

HOME REMEDIES
- Put sulfur or cayenne pepper in your socks.
- Mullein leaf tea

FEET, FEELING OF DEADNESS

HOME REMEDIES
- Bathe feet in potato water.

FEET, PAINFUL

HOME REMEDIES
- Lemon juice: Add 3 tsps. of lemon juice (or vinegar or boric acid) to 1 quart of water. Rinse your feet in this solution twice daily. It is supposed to help soothe and refresh sensitive skin.
- Tomatoes: Apply ripe, mashed to the soles of feet; or just apply a few slices. Bandage to feet and leave on all night. Soreness should be gone the next morning.

FEET, SWOLLEN

HOME REMEDIES
- Male fern root: Boil 2 ozs. fern in 3 quarts water for 30 minutes. Strain and let cool so it is comfortable to your feet. Bathe feet in it. Save liquid for the next day. Reduces morning swelling.
- Vinegar: Use vinegar water compresses for feet swollen at night.

FEMALE, BLEEDING

HOME REMEDIES

- Okra: Two tbls. cooked okra 3 times a day regulates female bleeding. You can get okra tablets in your health food store. Also good for general female complaints.
- Orange peeling tea: Used to stop female hemorrhages
- See your doctor.

FEMALE, TROUBLE (INFECTION) (SEE ALSO UTERUS)

HOME REMEDIES

- Nettle tea: Known for its antifungal and antiviral properties

FEVER

VITAMINS / MINERALS

- A, C, bioflavonoids, calcium lactate, trace minerals from raw potatoes

HOME REMEDIES

- In all fever diseases, there should be a fasting period of two days. Patient needs plenty of liquids, such as: diluted apple juice, diluted grape juice, herb tea with honey, cherry juice, fresh orange juice, lime and lemonade.
- Balm (*Melissa officinalis*) tea: 2 cups
- Coriander, marjoram, and willow bark teas

- Feverfew tea: 2 cups
- Garlic: In capsules
- Gentian: Cools the body and maintains digestive functions
- Herbal spice tea: Use equal parts cardamom, cloves, and a little black pepper.
- Lemon juice: Hot, with honey
- Pleurisy root reduces fever.

FEVER, BLISTERS

VITAMINS / MINERALS

- B_2

FEVER, CHILDREN

HOME REMEDIES

- Yellow jessamine (*Gelsemium sempervirens*) (homeopathic)
- *Echinacea angustifolia* (homeopathic)

FEVER, AND FLU

VITAMINS / MINERALS

- C

HOME REMEDIES

- Onion: Make an onion soup. This soup will bring vitamin C to work.

FEVERISH FEELING (SEE ALSO HEADACHE)

HOME REMEDIES
- Ginger, black pepper, honey

FEVER, TICK

HOME REMEDIES
- Chaparral: Take 3 tablets 3 times daily for one month.

FIBROID TUMOR

HOME REMEDIES
- Goldenrod tea
- Calendula (2 parts), yarrow (1 part), nettle (1 part): Mix and drink 1 quart daily for 4 weeks.

FINGER, PAIN (ACUTE)

HOME REMEDIES
- St. John's wort (*Hypericum perforatum*)

FINGER, SWOLLEN

HOME REMEDIES
- Iodine herbs

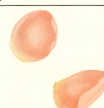

FINGERNAILS, CHEWING HABIT

VITAMINS / MINERALS
- Calcium

HOME REMEDIES
- Carrots and cauliflower are calcium-rich foods.

FINGERNAILS, RIDGED

HOME REMEDIES
- Silicon herbs

FINGERNAILS, SPLIT

VITAMINS / MINERALS
- Sulfur

FINGERNAILS, THIN

VITAMINS / MINERALS
- Sulfur

FLATULENCE (SEE ALSO HYSTERICAL FLATULENCE)

HOME REMEDIES
- Dill, anise, star anise: Equal parts, make tea.

FLU

VITAMINS / MINERALS

- Vitamin C for prevention

HOME REMEDIES

- Cayenne helps prevent colds/flu.
- Garlic and onion: Stimulate production of a detoxifying enzyme
- Grapefruit: Freshly squeezed grapefruit diluted with water. Equal parts water and grapefruit juice will ease the flu.
- Lettuce leaves: Take leaf lettuce and boil it in plenty of water. Drink 6 ozs. every hour.
- Oranges contain vitamin C.
- Red onion soup: Cut 1 large yellow onion in small pieces; cover with 2 quarts water; simmer for 1/2 hour. Strain and add honey to taste. Drink 2 cups every 2 hours until flu is gone.

FOOD, POISONING

HOME REMEDIES

- Ginger tea with honey: Drink.
- Vinegar: Take 2 tsps. apple cider vinegar in 1 glass water (no honey) and sip. Repeat every hour until all signs of food poisoning are gone.
- In case of severe vomiting: Moisten cloth with warm vinegar and apply to abdomen.
- For botulism: Combine 6 parts pokeroot and 3 parts sarsaparilla; make strong tea. Take 1/2 tbl. every 1/2 hour.

FRECKLES

HOME REMEDIES

- Lemon: Rub with a few drops of lemon.

FROSTBITE

VITAMINS / MINERALS

- K2 from alfalfa, niacin

HOME REMEDIES

- Lentils: Use as compress.
- Calamus root: Soak in calamus root tea.

FUNGUS

HOME REMEDIES

- Fungus grows in an alkaline medium. Natural antibiotics are grapefruit, garlic, willow, radish, chlorophyll, and bee pollen.
- Asparagus: Take 2 tbls. twice daily.
- Concord grape juice: Drink 3 glasses daily.

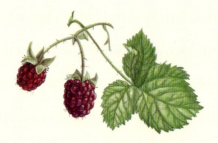

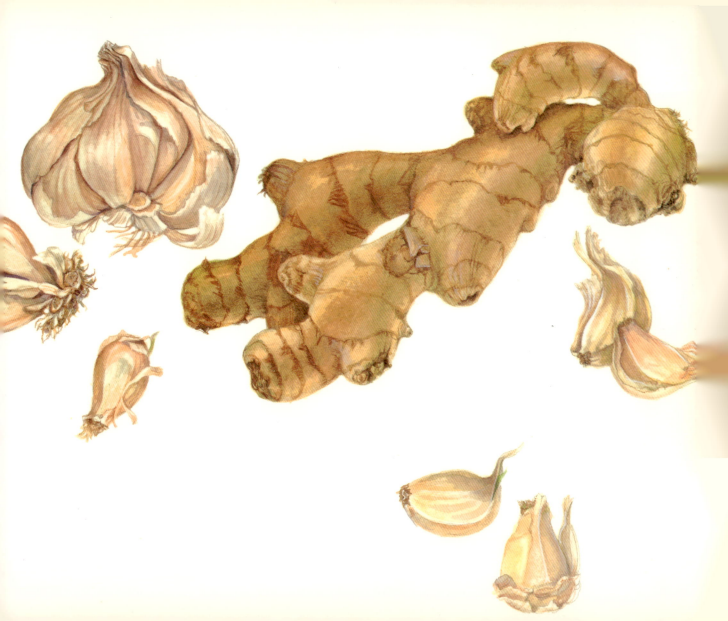

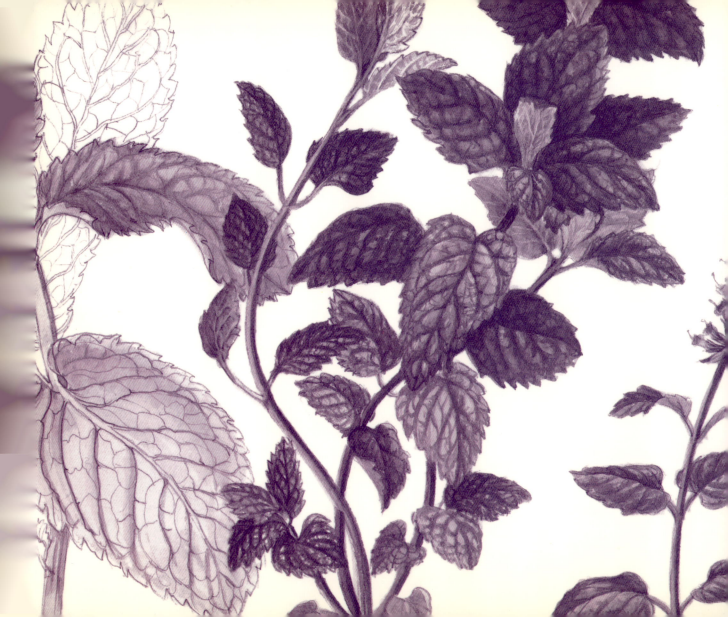

GALLBLADDER

HOME REMEDIES

- Artichoke: Increases flow of bile
- Lemon juice: Fresh lemon juice in 1 cup of hot water taken first thing in the morning will empty your gallbladder and start the day on a happy schedule. Two tsps. of lemon juice before each meal will strengthen the gallbladder.
- Radishes: Insufficient bile output can be aided by eating one small red radish (or white) before each meal.
- Pumpkin seeds: Take 1 heaping tsp. ground pumpkin seeds, cover with 7 ozs. of hot water, and drink slowly. Two cups a day are needed.
- Horseradish: Raw or dried will aid gallbladder.

GALLBLADDER, CHRONIC TROUBLE, OBSTRUCTIONS, OR PAIN

HOME REMEDIES

- Celandine (*Chelidonium majus*) (homeopathic)

GALLSTONES

HOME REMEDIES

- First day:
- 8 A.M. — 1 glass (18 oz.) apple juice
- 10 A.M. — 2 glasses (16 oz.) apple juice
- 12 NOON — 2 glasses (16 oz.) apple juice
- 2 P.M. — 2 glasses (16 oz.) apple juice
- 4 P.M. — 2 glasses (16 oz.) apple juice
- 6 P.M. — 2 glasses (16 oz.) apple juice
(Juice should be natural, without chemicals.)
- *Second day:* Same procedure as the first day. No food. At bedtime, 4 ozs. olive oil. You may wash the olive oil down with hot lemon juice.
- Black radish, olive oil: Take 2 tbls. grated black radish blended with 1 tbl. olive oil. Take 20 minutes before meals for gallstones.

GANGRENE

HOME REMEDIES

- Echinacea: In capsules
- Tomatoes: Raw, mashed tomatoes every 2 hours over the gangrene, then 1 hour rest. Leave on all night.
- Tobacco leaves: Poultice of tobacco leaves crushed (heals in 10 days)
- Willow leaves: Apply directly as a compress.

GAS, IN STOMACH AND INTESTINES

VITAMINS / MINERALS

- Sodium, magnesium

GAS, PAIN

HOME REMEDIES
- Allspice relieves gas.
- Certo: Add to ½ glass of apple juice and drink as needed.
- Rue tea: 1 cup with meals. (Do Not Use During Pregnancy.)

GASTRIC INDIGESTION

HOME REMEDIES
- Copper herbs

GASTRIC ULCER

HOME REMEDIES
- Cabbage: Very useful because it contains vitamin U.
- Cabbage juice: Freshly made cabbage juice, 6 ozs. before meals
- Carrots: Nothing to eat but cooked carrots for 7 days
- Potato juice: Freshly made potato juice, 7 ozs. between meals
- Potato soup made with milk

GASTRIC UPSET

HOME REMEDIES
- Arrowroot: Take 1 tsp. of arrowroot, make a smooth paste with cold milk or water, stir well, and boil. Add a little lime juice just before taking it.

GASTRITIS (INFLAMMATION OF STOMACH LINING)

VITAMINS / MINERALS
- A, B-complex from rice polishings, E, F, lecithin, trace minerals from flaxseed tea

HOME REMEDIES
- Flaxseed tea

GINGIVITIS

VITAMINS / MINERALS
- C, bioflavonoids

GLANDS, BALANCER

HOME REMEDIES
- Mallow leaf tea: Drink 2 cups daily.

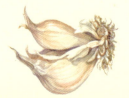

GLANDS, ENLARGED

VITAMINS / MINERALS
- Iodine, C, B-complex, F, pantothenic acid, lettuce water for trace minerals

GLANDS, SWOLLEN

HOME REMEDIES
- Watercress: Juice, 1 tbl. 5 times daily.
- Salad, eaten with a slice of buttered toast
- Marjoram
- Plantain leaves: Make an oil with these and apply. Plantain neutralizes poisons. Or boil and mix with salt; then use as a compress.
- Tomato: Place slice on swelling.
- Fenugreek seeds: Crush and combine with hot milk. Use as a poultice.

GLAUCOMA

VITAMINS / MINERALS
- A, B-complex, B2, C, bioflavonoids, E

HOME REMEDIES
- Restrict sweets as your physician tells you to.
- Yellow onion: Take a thin slice of yellow onion and hold over closed eyes. When tears come, take onion away and wash eyes in fresh, cold water. Do this every day for several weeks. No sugar of any kind if you have glaucoma.

GOITER

VITAMINS / MINERALS
- A, B-complex, calcium, kelp

HOME REMEDIES
- Agar-agar: 1 tsp. twice daily. Also, cool compresses overnight.
- Pokeroot tea: Drink 2 cups daily.

GONORRHEA

HOME REMEDIES
- Black walnut tea: 4 cups daily

GOUT

VITAMINS / MINERALS
- B-complex, C, E, pantothenic acid, sour cherries for minerals

HOME REMEDIES
- Onion: Make raw onion poultice over afflicted area. Leave it on all night.
- Hydrangea root tea: 2 cups daily.
- Comfrey root tea: 3 times daily.

GOUT AND STONE REMEDY

HOME REMEDIES
- Combine 1 quart apple cider, 1 tsp. hydrangea root: Let these stand for 12 hours, bring to a boil, simmer. Take 1/2 cup 3 times daily.

- Sour cherries: Take one small dish of sour cherries every morning for 3 weeks.

GRIEF, APPREHENSION

VITAMINS / MINERALS
- Magnesium
HOME REMEDIES
- Borage

GUM DISEASE

HOME REMEDIES
- Blue verrain (*Verbena hastata*) tea: Make strong and hold a small portion in mouth several times daily.
- Parsley tea: Use as above.
- Epsom salts: Hold a weak solution of Epsom salts in your mouth.
- Mulberry: Take 2-oz. twigs and cut into small pieces. Boil in 1 qt. white grape juice for 30 minutes. Cool, take 1 tbl. every 2 hours. Swish in mouth before swallowing.

GUMS, SORE

HOME REMEDIES
- Hyssop tea: Hold in mouth several times daily.

HAIR

VITAMINS / MINERALS
- A, B-complex, F, kelp for trace minerals

HAIR, BRITTLE

VITAMINS / MINERALS
- A
HOME REMEDIES
- Nettle tea: Wash hair with it.

HAIR, COLORING

HOME REMEDIES
- Nettle leaves

HAIR, DANDRUFF (WHITE, SCALY)

HOME REMEDIES
- Nettle; willow leaf tea

HAIR, DULL

VITAMINS / MINERALS
- Sulfur

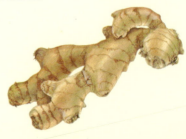

Hair, falling out

VITAMINS / MINERALS

- Sodium

HOME REMEDIES

- Could be a sign of an underactive thyroid. Eat high protein, no sugar at all, and plenty of yogurt.

Hair, graying

VITAMINS / MINERALS

- C, E, B-complex, folic acid, B12, PABA, pantothenic acid, copper, kelp

HOME REMEDIES

- Iodine herbs: To retain natural color

Hair, loss

HOME REMEDIES

- Nettle tea: drink
- Sarsaparilla
- Wormwood tea: Drink and rinse with cooled tea. Brew 2 tbls. in 1 quart of water for 25 minutes. Cool before moistening the scalp.
- Silicon herbs
- Could be a sign of underactive thyroid; eat high protein with no sugar at all and plenty of yogurt

Hair, loss (preventive)

HOME REMEDIES

- Rosemary: 1 pint of boiling water over 1 ounce of rosemary; mix into solution of 2 tbls. baking soda, strain and use as a hair rinse to prevent premature baldness.
- Thyme tea: Prevents or stops hair loss

Hair, oily

VITAMINS / MINERALS

- B2

HOME REMEDIES

- Wild hops

Hair, tonic

HOME REMEDIES

- Nettle tea

Halitosis

VITAMINS / MINERALS

- B-complex, choline, inositol, chlorophyll

HOME REMEDIES

- Chew juniper berries, caraway seed, or parsley leaves.
- Rosemary tea: Gargle.

HANGOVER

HOME REMEDIES

- Borage, thyme tea, cucumber: All help relieve a hangover.
- Fennel tea: Make, strain, and put in bathwater to detoxify the body and release toxic waste.

HAY FEVER

VITAMINS / MINERALS

- A, B-complex, C, pantothenic acid, sodium

HOME REMEDIES

- Carrots: Cut 3 carrots and cover with 1 quart water and boil for 20 minutes. Drink this broth as an exchange for the vegetable broth suggested.
- Vegetable broth: Every half hour drink 4 ozs. of pure water. Do this for 2 days. Then make yourself a vegetable broth and drink on the full hour 6 ozs. of broth and on the half hour 4 ozs. of water.
- Clover tea, red onion soup, and spikenard tea relieve hay fever.
- Wild plum tree bark: 2 ozs. to 1 quart of water. Boil down to 1 cup, add 1 cup of honey or maple or brown sugar and boil down again. Take 1 tbl. 4 times daily or as needed.
- Cherry bark tea: 2 cups daily

HAY FEVER, WITH ASTHMA

HOME REMEDIES

- Damask rose: 2 tbls. 4 times daily

HAY FEVER, WITH PROFUSE, YELLOW DISCHARGE

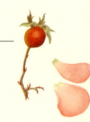

HOME REMEDIES

- Fenugreek
- Nettle tea

HEADACHE

HOME REMEDIES

- Nerve root (lady's slipper) tea
- Lavender: Applied hot will relieve almost any local pain. Also drink as a tea.
- Lavender oil: Applied to temples
- Brazilian cocoa (guarana) tea: 1 cup when headache starts
- Marjoram reduces headache.

HEADACHE, BACK OF HEAD

VITAMINS / MINERALS

- Potassium
- Might indicate liver or gallbladder trouble

HEADACHE, DULL

VITAMINS / MINERALS

- Iodine

HEADACHE, FRONT OF HEAD

HOME REMEDIES

- Might indicate kidney or bladder trouble

HEADACHE, LEFT SIDE OF HEAD

HOME REMEDIES

- Alfalfa tablets

HEADACHE, MIDDLE OF HEAD

HOME REMEDIES

- Indicates intestinal trouble

HEADACHE, MIGRAINE (SEE MIGRAINE)

HEADACHE, ON ONE SIDE OF HEAD

HOME REMEDIES

- Allergic reaction to something
- Allspice: Crush, take ½ ½ tsp. in juice twice daily.

HEADACHE, RADIATING FROM ONE POINT

HOME REMEDIES

- Black tea: 1 cup
- Vinegar: Wet a handkerchief with half vinegar and half water.

HEADACHE, RIGHT SIDE OF HEAD

HOME REMEDIES

- Celandine (*Chelidonium majus*) tea: 1 cup daily
- Orange: Peel and eat ½ at a time.

HEADACHE, TOP OF HEAD

HOME REMEDIES

- Indicates intestinal trouble.

HEADACHE, WITH NAUSEA

HOME REMEDIES

- Blue flag (*Iris versicolor*) (homeopathic)

HEARING, DULL

VITAMINS / MINERALS

- Iron

HEARING, LOSS (HARD OF HEARING)

VITAMINS / MINERALS
- Manganese (preventative), zinc

HOME REMEDIES
- Beth root tea: 2 cups daily.
- Horseradish: 2 drops of fresh horseradish juice in each ear
- Try calendula or marigold.

HEARING, RHEUMATIC DEAFNESS

HOME REMEDIES
- Garlic oil: Drench some cotton with garlic oil and put into ear.
- Wood betony: 2 cups daily
- Mistletoe (*Viscum album*) (homeopathic)

HEARING, RINGING IN EAR

HOME REMEDIES
- Blue flag (*Iris versicolor*) (homeopathic)

HEARING, SHRILL (HIGH-PITCHED)

HOME REMEDIES
- Violet leaf tea: 2 cups daily

HEART, ATTACK

HOME REMEDIES
- Compresses to the heart with vinegar water until physician arrives

HEART, BROKEN

HOME REMEDIES
- Poplar (balm of Gilead) buds: Carried in pocket or as tea

HEART, ENLARGED

VITAMINS / MINERALS
- B_1

HOME REMEDIES
- Asparagus: Take 2 tbls. 2 times daily.

HEART, EXTRA BEATS OR TOO FAST

VITAMINS / MINERALS
- B_1

HEART, FIBRILLATION

HOME REMEDIES
- Rosemary tea
- Chew on basil herb or cinnamon sticks.
- Lemon juice with cloves.

- Cool water: Put on face.

HEART, IRREGULARITY

VITAMINS / MINERALS
- Biotin

HOME REMEDIES
- Chew basil or cinnamon pieces.
- Rosemary tea; lemon water with cloves
- Basil tea or in capsules
- See your physician.

HEART, NERVOUS PALPITATION

VITAMINS / MINERALS
- B-complex, B6, lecithin, magnesium, calcium, and trace minerals from valerian root

HOME REMEDIES
- Rue tea (Not During Pregnancy)

HEART, PAIN (IRREGULARITY)

HOME REMEDIES
- Chew basil or cinnamon pieces; rosemary tea; lemon water with cloves.
- See your physician.

HEART, PALPITATIONS

HOME REMEDIES
- Cloves: Boil cloves in fresh or frozen lemon juice. Take 1 tsp. in 4 ozs. of water several times daily.

HEART, STRENGTHENER

HOME REMEDIES
- Cowslip (2 parts), lavender (1 part): Make tea using 1 tsp. per cup and drink 2 to 3 cups daily.

HEART, WEAKNESS (SLOW PULSE)

HOME REMEDIES
- Take 1 quart of water, add 2 tbls. vinegar. Wet a small towel and apply over chest close to the heart. Cover with woolen cloth. Change every hour. Results after several hours.

HEART, WEAKNESS OR ACHES (OR WHEN OVERWORKED)

HOME REMEDIES
- Parsley wine: Ten long-stemmed parsley, cut into 1/2-inch pieces (leaves and stems are used), cover with 1 quart natural white wine. Add 1 tbl. apple cider vinegar and bring to a boil. Simmer for 10 minutes, then add 3/4 cup of honey. Boil again for 5 more minutes. Strain wine and pour into hot, sterile bottles. Close tightly or set in refrigerator.

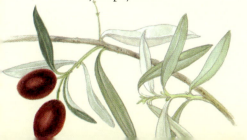

(*Caution*: Wine will run over easily while heating; stay with it.) Take 3 tbls. 2 to 3 times daily.

HEARTBURN

HOME REMEDIES

- Ginger: Take right after eating. Start with a small amount and work up to the right dosage for you.
- Slippery elm tea
- Potato: Eat a slice of raw potato when you have heartburn.

HEMORRHOIDS

VITAMINS / MINERALS

- B6, calcium, chlorophyll

HOME REMEDIES

- Almonds: Eat 3 a day to prevent and eliminate hemorrhoids.
- Stone root (*Collinsonia canadensis*) tea, or in capsules
- Dandelion root tea: Brew 15 minutes and drink 2 cups daily.
- Garlic: Oil a clove and insert it into the rectum each night for several nights in a row.
- Ginger tea: Relieves hot and painful hemorrhoids.
- Cranberries: Make a poultice; place over external hemorrhoids

- Sage: Make a pillow, fill with sage leaves, and keep it in place overnight.
- Potato: Slice and dip in oil to lubricate and insert into rectum.

HEPATITIS, INFECTIOUS

HOME REMEDIES

- Calendula (marigold) tea: With fresh lemon juice and distilled water. Add honey to taste. Drink 1 quart or more daily for 1 week. No fried foods or alcohol and keep warm.

HERNIA

HOME REMEDIES

- Mistletoe, horsetail: Combine and apply as poultice overnight.

HERPES, GENERAL

VITAMINS / MINERALS

- C, E, zinc, lysine (500 mg. once a day)

HOME REMEDIES

- Buck bean tea: 1 cup daily
- Club moss; Buttercup (*Ranunculus bulbosis*) (homeopathic)
- Olive leaf compound

HERPES II, BLISTER TYPE

HOME REMEDIES
- Buttercup (*Ranunculus bulbosis*)
  (homeopathic)
- Black walnut tea

HERPES, LABIALIS (WITH ITCHING/ SENSATION OF HEAT)

HOME REMEDIES
- Nettle tea

HERPES ZOSTER (SEE ALSO SHINGLES)

VITAMINS / MINERALS
- B-complex, chlorophyll, B1, magnesium, calcium
HOME REMEDIES
- Houseleek: In soup or salad
- Blue flag (*Iris versicolor*) (homeopathic)

HICCUPS

HOME REMEDIES
- Blow into a paper bag.
- Vinegar: A few drops on 1 tsp. of sugar.
  One spoonful in some water.
- Anise: Make 1 cup of anise tea and sip slowly.
- Orange: Cut in half; squeeze juice from
  1/2 orange into a glass and drink slowly. Repeat

with other half if necessary.
- Pineapple juice relieves hiccups.

HIP, PAIN (TO FEET)

HOME REMEDIES
- Cayenne pepper: Put in socks.

HIVES (SEE URTICARIA)

HOARSENESS (SEE ALSO LARYNGITIS)

HOME REMEDIES
- Drink ginger tea with honey.
- Plantain tea: Make it strong and sip.
  It neutralizes poison.
- Black bean juice: Take black beans and boil them
  in plenty of water (1 pound of beans to 1 gallon
  of water); boil for 1 hour, strain. Drink the juice,
  6 ozs., 3 to 4 times daily. Eat beans in another dish
  or in soup.
- Glycerin: 1 tbl. in hot water; gargle often

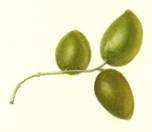

HOOKWORM

HOME REMEDIES

- Thyme tea: Two cups strong tea followed by a dose of Epsom salts. Take Epsom salts $1/2$ hour after the tea.

HORMONES, FEMALE

HOME REMEDIES

- Black cohosh, rice polishings
- Booster: $1/2$ cup ground cashews, 2 tbls. rice polishings, 2 cups water or apple juice. Blend in blender, add honey if wanted. Gives women charm and femininity.
- Supply: pumpkin seeds.

HORMONES, MALE

HOME REMEDIES

- Sarsaparilla, brewer's yeast
- Booster: 2 tbls. brewer's yeast; 1 tsp. chia seed, 1 cup cashews, 2 cups tomato juice. Blend in blender. Gives men willpower and determination.
- Supply: Pumpkin seeds.

HUMAN PAPILLOMA VIRUS

HOME REMEDIES

- Drink concord grape juice every day. Douche with concord grape juice as well.

HYDROCEPHALUS

HOME REMEDIES

- Hellebore tea: Take 1 tsp. 4 times daily.

HYPERACTIVE, CHILDREN

HOME REMEDIES

- Thyme tea: 2 cups daily, 1 tsp. to 1 cup
- Chem-x (homeopathic)

HYPER INSULINISM

VITAMINS / MINERALS

- A, B-complex, C, pantothenic acid, zinc, sulfur from hops tea

HYPERTENSION

HOME REMEDIES

- Onions: Contain a substance called prostaglandin. This is normally produced in the human body and is known to have an anti-hypertensive effect.

HYPOCHONDRIA

HOME REMEDIES
- Vanilla: Take 1 vanilla bean, cut in pieces. Boil it in 1 cup of water for 5 minutes. Sweeten with honey.
- Cherries: Eat morning and night for hypochondria.

HYPOGLYCEMIA

HOME REMEDIES
- Three drops sassafras oil in 1 tbl. fruit juice, twice daily for 4 weeks.
- Red beets help people with low blood sugar.

HYSTERIA

VITAMINS / MINERALS
- Sodium

HOME REMEDIES
- Passion flowers: 1 cup twice daily.
- Wood betony

HYSTERIA, CONNECTED WITH FEMALE TROUBLE

HOME REMEDIES
- Motherwort tea: Drink 1 cup twice daily.

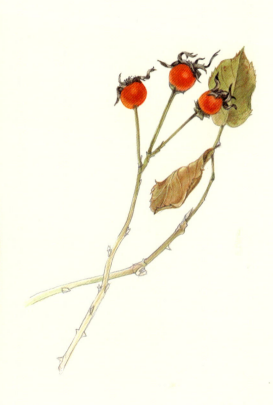

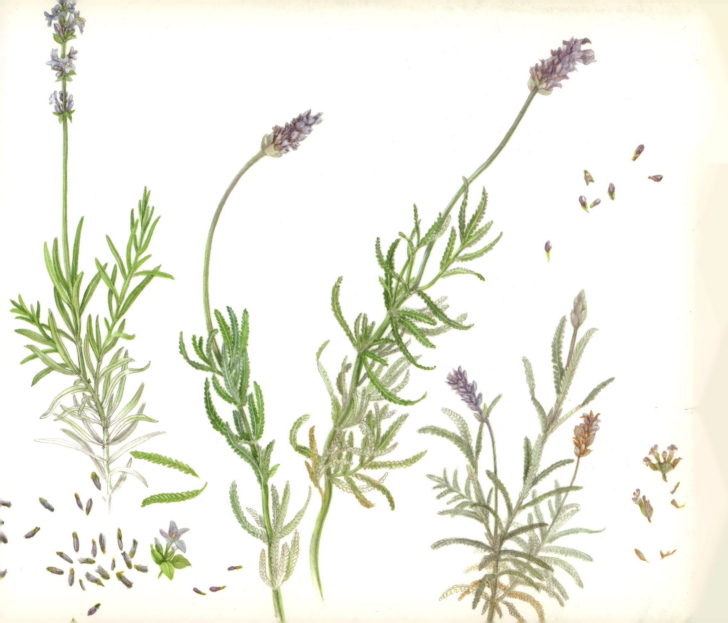

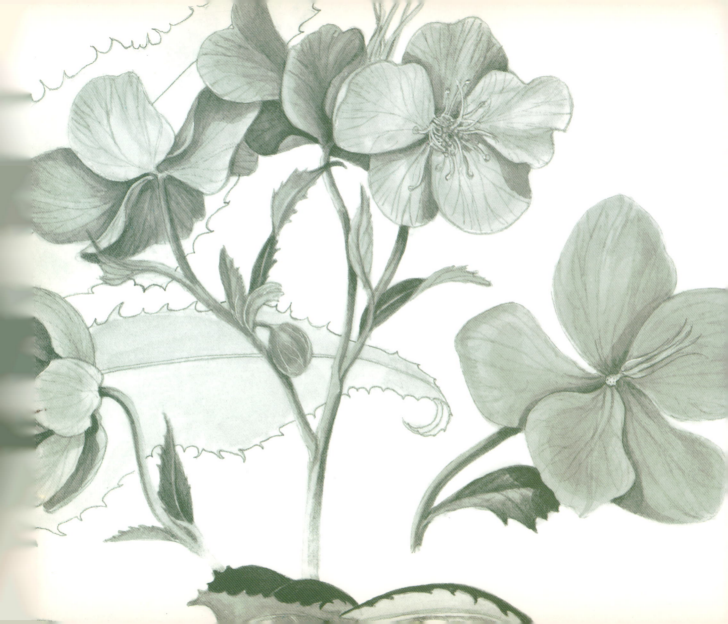

IMMUNE SYSTEM

HOME REMEDIES

- Take flaxseed and walnuts to stimulate the immune system. They contain alpha linoleic acid.

IMPETIGO (PUS-FILLED PIMPLES, ESPECIALLY OVER FACE AND SCALP)

VITAMINS / MINERALS

- A, E, folic acid

HOME REMEDIES

- Pansy tea and/or as a rinse

IMPOTENCE

HOME REMEDIES

- Fenugreek seed tablets

INDIGESTION

VITAMINS / MINERALS

- Sodium

HOME REMEDIES

Summer savory
- Citrus family: To 1 quart water add the juice of 1 grapefruit, 1 lemon, 3 oranges, 2 tbls. milk sugar, 1 cup aloe vera. Drink in small sips; 1 quart per day.

- Whey: 1 tbl. of whey in a little water helps digestion.
- Slippery elm tea (for chronic indigestion)

INFECTION

VITAMINS / MINERALS

- Take plenty of pantothenic acid when fighting an infection.

HOME REMEDIES

- Parsley, Black radish, Savory, Basil: Used to treat infections
- Cranberries: Boil and use juice to fight infections.
- Grapefruit: Finely grated skin of 1 grapefruit. Take 1 tsp. and add juice of 1/2 grapefruit. Drink 3 times daily to fight infection.

INFECTION, LOW GRADE

VITAMINS / MINERALS

- Sulfur

HOME REMEDIES

- Natural antibiotics: Garlic, grapefruit, chlorophyll, parsley and radish, willow, bee pollen extract
- Cranberries: Boil and use the juice.
- Potato: Suck raw potatoes and spit out the pulp. Or make 1 cup raw potato juice, add to 3 cups water, and drink.

INFECTION, SKIN

HOME REMEDIES

- White pond lily: Apply to skin.

INFECTION, TENDENCY TO

VITAMINS / MINERALS

- A, C, E, bioflavonoids, calcium lactate, minerals from fresh lemon juice

HOME REMEDIES

- Fresh lemon juice

INFECTION, VIRUS

HOME REMEDIES

- Calendula tea; Olive leaf compound

INFECTIOUS DISEASE, GENERAL (SEE ALSO PREVENTION, INFECTIOUS DISEASES)

HOME REMEDIES

- Warm milk compresses all over the body Wrap patient in first layer of warm milk sheet; second layer, woolen blanket; third layer, warm cover. Repeat in 2 hours if needed.

INFECTIOUS DISEASE, HEPATITIS

HOME REMEDIES

- Calendula (marigold)
- Fresh lime juice

INFECTIOUS DISEASE, LUNG

HOME REMEDIES

- Onions: Boil, mash, and place them between 2 layers of cloth. Apply to chest for about 2 hours.

INFECTIOUS DISEASE, SINUS

HOME REMEDIES

- Pepper and honey: Take 1 tsp. honey and sprinkle with freshly ground pepper. Also good for sniffles.

INFECTIOUS DISEASE, STAPH

HOME REMEDIES

- Grapefruit: Grate the skin of a grapefruit with a fine grater. Take 1 tsp. and add the juice of $1/2$ grapefruit. Drink this 3 times a day.

INFLAMMATION

HOME REMEDIES

- Flaxseed, soy products, purslane, and walnuts all reduce inflammation.
- Fenugreek: Add crushed seeds to hot milk and make poultice.

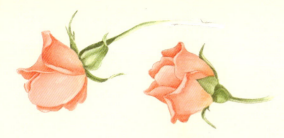

- Inflammation of body may point to protozoan infection. Take specific homeopathic remedies to help relieve inflammation.

INFLAMMATION, COLON

HOME REMEDIES
- Irish potato peel and flaxseed meal: Make tea.

INFLAMMATION, EYE AND EYELID

HOME REMEDIES
- Elder flower (externally). Also, drink 2 cups a day.
- Use raw potato poultice over eye.

INFLAMMATION, LIPS AND MOUTH

VITAMINS / MINERALS
- B6, niacin

INFLAMMATION, MUSCLES

VITAMINS / MINERALS
- C, E, pantothenic acid

IINFLUENZA

VITAMINS / MINERALS
- A, C, B-complex, pantothenic acid, minerals from linden blossom tea and mint tea
- Linden blossom and mint teas

INJURIES, BONE, TENDON, AND MUSCLE

HOME REMEDIES
- Comfrey root compresses

INJURIES, DEEPER TISSUE

HOME REMEDIES
- Daisy tea: Drink 2 to 3 cups daily.

INJURIES, NERVES

HOME REMEDIES
- Daisy tea: Drink 2 to 3 cups daily.

INJURIES, SINEW, TENDON, AND JOINT

HOME REMEDIES
- Comfrey root compresses
- Arnica is best.

JOINTS, PAIN

VITAMINS / MINERALS

- Sulfur
- Comfrey root tea: Apply and drink.
- Comfrey root tincture: Apply.
- Combine: Avocado seeds (chopped) and horsetail grass (3 oz.). Boil together in 1 quart water, down to 1 pint. Add rubbing alcohol; use as liniment.
- Simmer laurel beans in any oil and apply over aching joints.

JOINTS, STIFF

VITAMINS / MINERALS

- Use manganese for joint cracking.

HOME REMEDIES

- Cabbage: Raw poultice. Grate 2 cups very fine, wrap in cheesecloth, and apply overnight. For best results, do it several nights in a row.
- Cucumber: The natural sodium makes joints limber.
- Olive leaf compound

JOINTS, SWOLLEN

HOME REMEDIES

- Extract potato juice and boil to $^1/_5$ original amount. Add glycerin to preserve it. Make poultice.

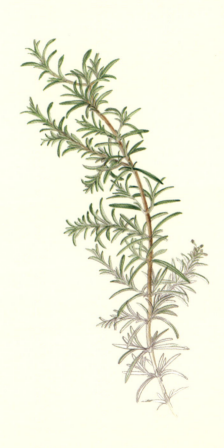

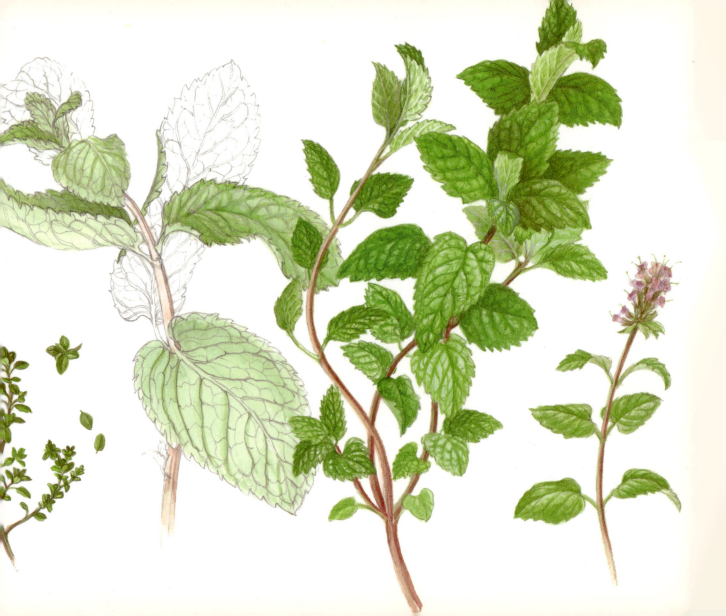

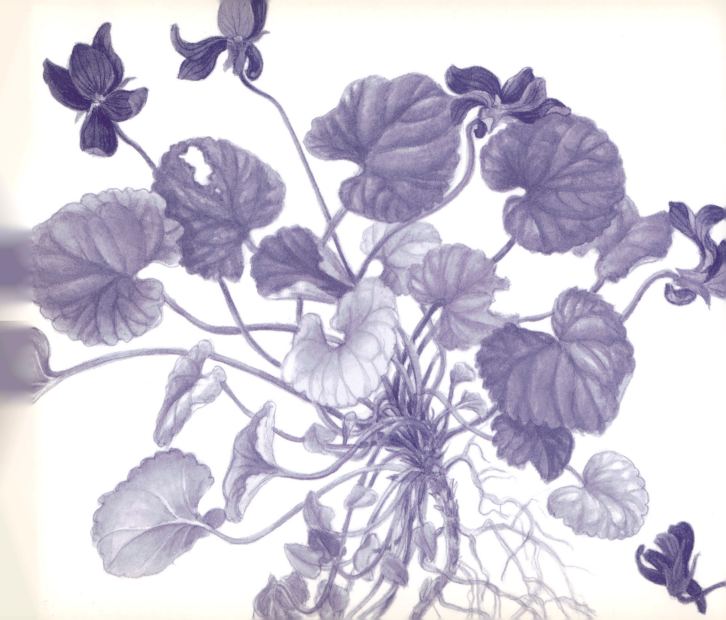

KIDNEYS

VITAMINS / MINERALS

- A, B-complex, C, magnesium, trace minerals from herb teas

HOME REMEDIES

- Herb teas: Watermelon seed, couchgrass, cornsilk, uva ursi
- Cranberry juice: Drink plenty every day.
- Cinnamon warms the kidneys.
- Cold pressed oils are needed to assimilate the proteins from vegetables. They are food to the kidney.

KIDNEYS, AND/OR BLADDER STONES

VITAMINS / MINERALS

- A, B-complex, stone root tea for minerals (for kidney stones)

HOME REMEDIES

- Anise: Put 1 tbl. in 1 quart grape juice and simmer for 1/2 hour. Drink 7 oz. 3 times daily.
- Parsley tea: Drink for 3 days with no other food.
- Asparagus: Dissolves oxalic acid crystals when they are lodged in the kidneys.
- Grape juice (dark): 1 cup or 7 ozs., add 1/2 tsp. cream of tartar. Take 2 ozs. 3 times daily before meals.

- Dandelion root: Boil 2 tbls. in 1 quart apple juice for 10 minutes. Strain and drink 6 ozs. 3 times daily (for kidney stones).
- Beets: Boil 5 whole, medium-sized beets in 3 quarts of water for 1 hour. Drink 7 ozs. of the water 3 times daily.
- Use cucumber juice or tea from avocado leaf. Or take brown corn water—allow to steep, then drink 1 cup daily (diuretic for kidney stones).
- Chamomile and knotgrass (for kidney stones)

KIDNEYS, AND/OR BLADDER TROUBLE

HOME REMEDIES

- Celery tops: Eat after each meal for 5 weeks.

KIDNEYS, BLEEDING

VITAMINS / MINERALS

- Choline: Is a methyl donor and increases the metabolism in general and liver and kidney in particular

HOME REMEDIES

- Watermelon seed tea

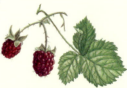

KIDNEYS, CATARRHAL (INFLAMMATION) (SEE ALSO BRIGHT'S DISEASE)

HOME REMEDIES

- Juniper berries
- Watermelon and seeds: For 2 days, eat nothing but watermelon. Always eat the melon by itself.
- Indian remedy: One radish 3 times a day

KIDNEYS, CONGESTION

HOME REMEDIES

- Blue vervain (*Verbena hastata*) tea

KIDNEYS, DYSFUNCTION

HOME REMEDIES

- Asparagus: Boil in plenty of water (2 quarts water to 4 ozs. asparagus) and use the concoction, 1 cup, 4 times daily. Strongly diuretic in action.
- Horseradish boiled in apple juice gives copious urine if kidney is blocked.

KIDNEYS, INFECTION

HOME REMEDIES

- Watermelon: Eat all you want for 2 days; no other food.

KIDNEYS, TROUBLE

HOME REMEDIES

- Cranberry juice: Combine 1/2 cranberry juice, 1/2 water. Take 7 oz. 3 times daily.

LABOR, PAIN

VITAMINS / MINERALS

- B1, calcium lactate

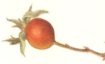

LABOR, PROLONGED

VITAMINS / MINERALS

- B1

LABYRINTHITIS (INNER EAR)

VITAMINS / MINERALS

- C, bioflavonoids, B-complex, B12, folic acid, E

LACTATION

HOME REMEDIES

- Anise can enhance milk production and relieve bloated conditions in nursing child.
- Caraway seeds: Increase mother's milk Add 1 tsp. seeds to 8 oz. cold water. Bring to boil and simmer for a few minutes. Drink several cups a day.
- Dill tea: Increases mother's milk

- Fennel tea: Promotes lactation and relieves colic in nursing child
- Lentils and borage are good for lactation.

LACTATION, INCREASE IN MILK

HOME REMEDIES
- Blessed thistle tea

LACTATION, INCREASE IN QUALITY

HOME REMEDIES
- Alfalfa tea

LARYNGITIS (SEE ALSO HOARSENESS)

HOME REMEDIES
- Arnica tincture: 3 to 4 drops in 1 tbl. warm water several times daily
- Violet leaf tea: Drink or gargle.
- Black beans: Juice is good for hoarseness and laryngitis.
- Red onions relieve laryngitis.

LARYNGITIS, CHRONIC

HOME REMEDIES
- *Thuja occidentalis* (homeopathic)

LARYNX, TICKLING

HOME REMEDIES
- Red onion: Raw or as soup

LAXATIVE

HOME REMEDIES
- Prunes, apricots: Mix 3 prunes and 3 apricots. Soak overnight and take this much twice daily. This combination is special.

LEGS, CRAMPS

VITAMINS / MINERALS
- Calcium (for cramps at night);
- Calcium when left leg hurts; magnesium when right leg hurts.
- Potassium

HOME REMEDIES
- Club moss (*Lycopodium clavatum*): Wrap as a compress, put in a pillow, or use in homeopathic form.
- Cramp bark tea
- Male fern: Foot baths
- Eat more fruit.
- Homeopathic: *Arsenicum album*

LEGS, SWOLLEN

HOME REMEDIES
- Lady's mantle

LEUKEMIA

VITAMINS / MINERALS
- Shortage of zinc: Chlorophyll from watermelon rind and seeds

HOME REMEDIES
- Sulfur herbs
- Okra: Gives strength
- Red beets: Valuable factors contribute substantially to the health of the body.
- Watermelon rind and seeds
- In all cases, the tailbone should be checked and realigned.

LEUKOPENIA (DIMINISHING OF WHITE BLOOD CORPUSCLES)

VITAMINS / MINERALS
- B6

LICE

HOME REMEDIES
- Mineral oil: Warm; pour over entire scalp. After 10 minutes, shampoo. Then use a fine-toothed comb to gather the suffocated lice. Repeat

procedure every 2 days for 10 days.
- Thyme tea: Use as a skin antiseptic.

LIVER

VITAMINS / MINERALS
- A, C, E, potassium, choline, inositol

HOME REMEDIES
- Apricots, pineapple juice: Use to detoxify liver and pancreas. Soak 1 pound dried apricots in pineapple juice. Next morning, blend mixture. Take this 2 days in a row.
- Casaba melon: Take by itself.
- Carrot juice: 6 oz. with 2 tbls. cream, taken 1 hour after breakfast
- Combine: $1/2$ quart carrot juice, $1/2$ quart goat's milk, 1 tbl. molasses per quart
- Also, white beans, artichokes, allspice, and apples are helpful.

LIVER, AILMENT

HOME REMEDIES
- Breakfast: 2 tbls. ground flaxseed, 2 tbls. whey, 2 peeled and finely grated apples. Mix and serve with honey. Healing to the liver and intestines.

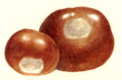

LIVER, CIRRHOSIS

VITAMINS / MINERALS
- Selenium

HOME REMEDIES
- Club moss compresses

LIVER, CLEANSER

HOME REMEDIES
- Chaparral tea or capsules

LIVER, CONGESTION

HOME REMEDIES
- Blue vervain (*Verbena hastata*) tea:
  2 cups daily

LIVER, CONSTIPATION DUE TO

HOME REMEDIES
- Barberry tea: 1 cup with meals

LIVER, DAMAGE

HOME REMEDIES
- Dandelion leaves and stems (not the flowers)

LIVER, ENLARGED

HOME REMEDIES
- Dandelion tea; or fresh salads
- Flaxseed: Place in a little bag, hang it in boiling hot water for 10 minutes. Squeeze excess water out and apply over liver area. Cover with a towel.

LIVER STRENGTHENER

HOME REMEDIES
- Dandelion root tea

LIVER, SWOLLEN

HOME REMEDIES
- Potato: Cook red potatoes, mash them, place between two layers of cloth, and apply warm to the liver.
- Goldenrod, goldenseal root, cloves (herbal formula)
- Lime juice: Fresh squeezed from 2 limes, combined with distilled water (1 quart), and honey to taste. Drink 1 quart or more daily for 7 days. Do not chill. Drink at room temperature. Do not eat any fried foods or alcoholic beverages, and keep your feet warm.

LIVER/PANCREAS

HOME REMEDIES

- Nutmeg: Add 1/2 tsp. to 1 cup hot water; acts as a stimulant.
- Apricots detoxify liver/pancreas.

LOW BLOOD PRESSURE (SEE BLOOD PRESSURE, LOW)

LOW BLOOD SUGAR

VITAMINS / MINERALS

- Iron herbs, ferric phosphate (cell salt #4)

HOME REMEDIES

- Oil of sassafras: Rub in 3 drops on the sole of each foot twice daily for 4 weeks.

LUMBAGO

VITAMINS / MINERALS

- B-complex, B1

LUNG, ABSCESSES

HOME REMEDIES

- Cucumber juice

LUNG, CONGESTION

HOME REMEDIES

- Fenugreek relieves congestion.
- Thyme tea: Relieves shortness of breath
- Water: Aerate pure water by beating it with an eggbeater. Drink it at once.

LUNG, COUGH (PHLEGM)

HOME REMEDIES

- Lungwort tea: 1 to 4 cups daily

LUNG, DISEASES

HOME REMEDIES

- Cabbage is anti-inflammatory and antibacterial.
- Cardamom has a soothing effect on membranes and lungs.
- Add dill to your food. Eat fish, vegetables, salads, very few carbohydrates, and lots of cream, fat, or butter.

LUNG, STRENGTHENER

HOME REMEDIES

- Calamus root

LUNG, WEAK

HOME REMEDIES

- Lungwort tea: 1 to 4 cups daily

LUPUS (SKIN)

HOME REMEDIES

- *Thuja occidentalis* (homeopathic)
- Bring wine vinegar to a boil and thicken it with barley flour. Apply to skin.

LYMPH GLANDS, DISEASED

HOME REMEDIES

- Echinacea: 2 capsules or more daily for 3 days

LYMPH GLANDS, ENLARGED

HOME REMEDIES

- Pokeroot tea

LYMPH GLANDS, SWOLLEN

HOME REMEDIES

- Lettuce; basil

LYMPHATIC SYSTEM

VITAMINS / MINERALS

- Potassium

HOME REMEDIES

- Cucumber: 4 or 5 cups of cucumber juice a day for 1 week purifies the lymphatic system and the blood and clears the complexion.
- Bananas keep lymphatic system fit.

LYMPHATIC TROUBLE

HOME REMEDIES

- Burdock root tea: 2 cups daily

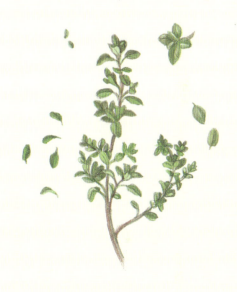

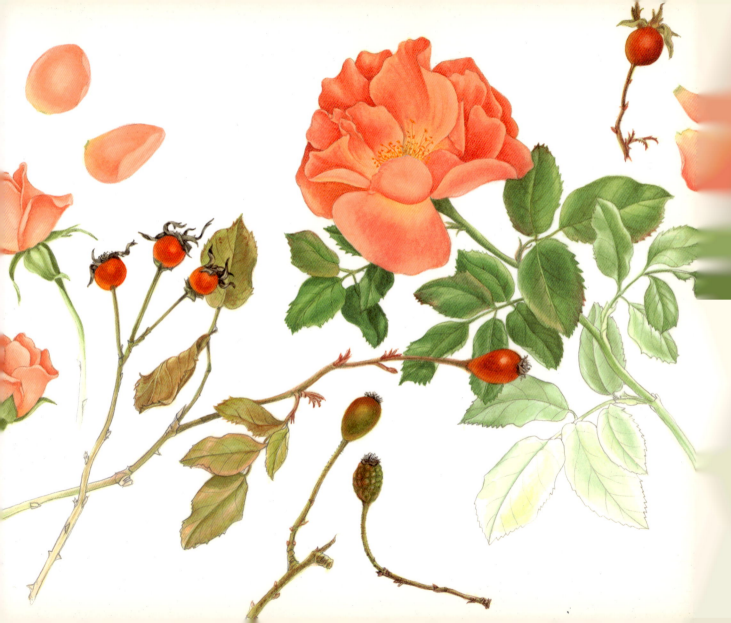

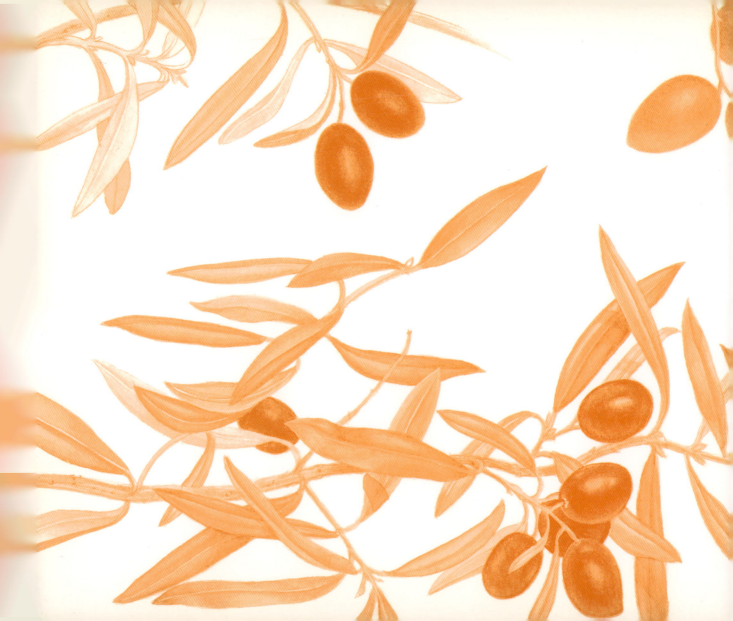

MALARIA

HOME REMEDIES

- Collard seed, parsley seed, red pepper seed

MAMMARY GLANDS, UNDERDEVELOPED

HOME REMEDIES

- Saw palmetto (Sabal serrulate) (homeopathic)

MEASLES

VITAMINS / MINERALS

- C, minerals from raw potatoes (grated)

HOME REMEDIES

- First stage: Eyebright
- Later stage: Wind flower (*Pulsatilla*) (homeopathic); Alfalfa seeds; Linden blossoms

MEMORY

HOME REMEDIES

- Almonds: Take 6 to 10 a day.
- Almond oil: Take 1 tsp. a day.
- Cloves: 4 cloves in any tea mixture, daily
- Eyebright tablets
- Mustard seeds: 2 seeds for memory
- Prunes: Take 3 daily.
- Rosemary tea
- Sage: On a slice of buttered rye bread
- Ginkgo biloba

MENIERS SYNDROME

VITAMINS / MINERALS

- B-complex, B6, B1, B12, C, E, F, niacin, potassium, bioflavonoids

MENINGITIS

HOME REMEDIES

- Aloe vera leaves: Take a couple, about 6 inches long, and wash and cut into small pieces. Add 3 times the amount of water and simmer for 10 minutes. Add 2 tbls. honey or more to taste and simmer for another 5 minutes. Cool, strain and give 1 tbl. to adult every hour, and 1 tsp. to a child every hour. The sicker you are, the smaller the dosage.
- Goldenseal, skullcap: Make tea to use for enemas.

MENOPAUSE

VITAMINS / MINERALS

- Calcium, magnesium, red bone marrow
- B-complex: A high potency taken 1 to 3 times daily further supports the nervous system, and a daily intake of vitamin E has been known to eliminate hot flashes and night sweats.
- Vitamin D: Needed in adequate amounts or a deficiency causes nervousness, irritability, and headaches. Depression and arthritic problems may develop.

HOME REMEDIES

- Black cohosh: In capsules
- Rue tea: 2 cups daily.
- Yarrow: In capsules
- Cinnamon; yams also beneficial.

MENSES, REGULATOR

HOME REMEDIES

- Wind flower (*Pulsatilla*) (homeopathic)

MENSTRUAL CRAMPS, RELIEVED

HOME REMEDIES

- Lemon balm, motherwort, oregano help relieve cramps.
- Cramp bark: 1 cup tea as needed

MENSTRUAL DIFFICULTIES

HOME REMEDIES

- Blue cohosh: 2 capsules needed

MENSTRUAL FLOW, EXCESSIVE

VITAMINS / MINERALS

- B-complex, B12, E, folic acid, iron, trace minerals from okra

HOME REMEDIES

- Okra
- Shepherd's purse tea: 2 cups daily

MENSTRUAL FLOW, IRREGULAR

VITAMINS / MINERALS

- B-complex, E, folic acid, sulfur, trace minerals from fireweed

MENSTRUAL FLOW, PROMOTES

HOME REMEDIES

- Motherwort tea
- Hot ginger tea: stimulates delayed menses; relieves cramps

MENSTRUAL FLOW, SCANTY

HOME REMEDIES

- Thyme tea

MENSTRUATION, CLOTS

HOME REMEDIES

- Shepherd's purse: 2 cups daily, 1 tsp. to 1 cup of boiling water

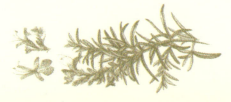

MENSTRUATION, DISTURBED DUE TO EMOTION

HOME REMEDIES
- Tiger Lily (*Lilium tigrinum*) (homeopathic)

MENSTRUATION, PMS (SEE PREMENSTRUAL SYNDROME)

MENTAL DEPRESSION

VITAMINS / MINERALS
- Sodium

HOME REMEDIES
- Cleavers tea

MENTAL HEALTH

HOME REMEDIES
- Iodine herbs

MENTAL INSTABILITY

HOME REMEDIES
- Agar, sorrel: Make tea and drink.

MIGRAINE (SEE ALSO HEADACHE)

HOME REMEDIES
- Blue vervain (*Verbena hastata*) tea
- At the start of a headache: Brazilian cocoa (guarana)
- Lavender oil: on forehead
- A specific homeopathic remedy for dioxin

MISCARRIAGE

HOME REMEDIES
- Rosemary can help prevent miscarriage.
- Apple tree bark tea will check miscarriages.

MONONUCLEOSIS

VITAMINS / MINERALS
- B-complex, B6, C, E, pantothenic acid, copper, trace minerals from lettuce water and raspberry leaf tea

HOME REMEDIES
- Red raspberry leaf tea
- Leaf lettuce water/tea
- Apply raw tomato poultices to the neck for swelling.

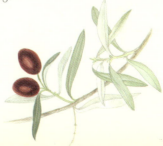

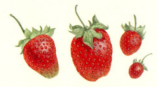

MORNING SICKNESS

VITAMINS / MINERALS

- B6 and trace minerals from peach leaf tea

HOME REMEDIES

- Peach leaf tea

MOSQUITO BITE

HOME REMEDIES

- Bar soap: Moisten a little and rub over bite. It will stop itching.
- Mix baking soda and cream of tartar with a bit of water to make a paste. Apply to bite.

MOUTH, BURNING

HOME REMEDIES

- Poppy seed (available in your spice section): Make tea. Hold in your mouth several times a day.

MOUTH, DRY

HOME REMEDIES

- Chew cloves or calamus root.

MOUTH, ODOR

HOME REMEDIES

- Juniper berries, caraway seed, or parsley leaves: Chew.
- Rosemary tea: Gargle.

MOUTH, ULCERS

VITAMINS / MINERALS

- Zinc (when corners of mouth are cracked)

HOME REMEDIES

- Chew sage or willow leaves.
- Hold blackberry leaf tea in mouth.
- Myrrh
- Carrots: Grated, wrapped in a cloth and applied to canker sores. Change every 2 hours.

MUCOUS

HOME REMEDIES

- Oranges: Cleansers of the stomach, ears, head, and sinuses if taken in the following manner: Drink 1 glass of fresh-squeezed juice followed by the same amount of distilled water. DO NOT MIX. Do this as often as you want, 10 times daily or so. NO OTHER FOODS should be taken for 2 days. Do this 2 days in a row, 3 times a year.

MUCOUS, SOLVENT

HOME REMEDIES
- Fenugreek; Southernwood
- In bronchi, rattling: Garlic
- In lungs: Calamus root tea

MULTIPLE SCLEROSIS

VITAMINS / MINERALS
- B-complex, E, C, B, B15, lecithin, niacin, magnesium, pantothenic acid

HOME REMEDIES
- Pineapple and avocado
- Thyme tea
- Make tea of sunflower and fenugreek seeds: Drink 1 cup 3 times daily.
- Combine corn, grated carrots, liquid garlic, chives, milk, dry mustard, paprika, flaxseed oil, and primrose oil. Place all in a blender; add salt or pepper to taste.
- Emu-mu drops help rebuild the central nervous system.

MUMPS

HOME REMEDIES
- Pokeroot tea: 1 cup 3 times daily
- Linden flower bath: Take a handful of flowers, brew, strain, and add to bath.

MUMPS, AFTER SECOND STAGE

HOME REMEDIES
- Wind flower (*Pulsatilla*) (homeopathic)
- Gotu kola
- Linden blossom tea

MUMPS, RESIDUE

HOME REMEDIES
- Gotu kola: In capsules

MUSCLE, ACHES IN SHOULDER

VITAMINS / MINERALS
- Magnesium

MUSCLE, BUILDERS

HOME REMEDIES
- Beans and corn: Use in various combinations, such as beans and corn bread or corn tortillas and beans.
- Rye

MUSCLE, CALVES VERY TENSE

HOME REMEDIES
- Chickpea (*Lathyrus sativus*) (homeopathic)

MUSCLE, CRAMPS

VITAMINS / MINERALS
- B1, B2, E, calcium lactate

MUSCLE, DETERIORATION

HOME REMEDIES
- Shepherd's purse tea: Drink 2 cups daily.

MUSCLE, FUNCTION

VITAMINS / MINERALS
- E

MUSCLE, JERKS

VITAMINS / MINERALS
- Magnesium needed

MUSCLE, PAIN

VITAMINS / MINERALS
- B, E, calcium lactate
HOME REMEDIES
- Rub a piece of raw potato over the muscle.

MUSCLE, SPASMS (DAYTIME)

VITAMINS / MINERALS
- Magnesium

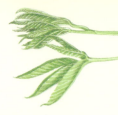

HOME REMEDIES
- Marjoram

MUSCLE, SPASMS (EVENING)

VITAMINS / MINERALS
- Calcium lactate
HOME REMEDIES
- Marjoram

MUSCLE, STRENGTH

HOME REMEDIES
- Buckwheat: Use in pancakes, cereal, or main dishes.
- Chia seed: Soak 1 tsp. seed in 4 ozs. of juice for 2 to 3 hours and drink this 3 to 4 times a day.

MUSCLE, TENDON AND TISSUE INJURIES

HOME REMEDIES
- Apply comfrey root compresses.
- Arnica tincture: A few drops in water, make compress. Also put a few drops in water and drink.
- Daisy tea: Drink 2 to 3 cups daily.
- Lady's mantle (*Alchemilla vulgaris*)

MUSCLE, TWITCHING

HOME REMEDIES
- Skullcap

MUSCLE, WEAKNESS

VITAMINS / MINERALS
- Potassium

HOME REMEDIES
- Apple peelings: Take a handful of peelings, boil them for 20 minutes in 1 quart water. Strain and take 6 ozs. daily.
- Jerusalem artichokes
- Sesame seeds: Complete amino acid supplier. Supplies osmium, a trace mineral.
- Shepherd's purse
- Gentian tea: $1/2$ cup twice daily.
- Wormwood with lady's mantle tea.

MUSCLE, WEAKNESS AFTER ILLNESS

HOME REMEDIES
- Almonds: Eat alone or add to food.

MUSCLE, WEAKNESS IN CHILDREN

HOME REMEDIES
- Barley malt
- Juniper berry branches: Boil for 45 minutes, strain, and add the tea to bathwater. Soak for 20 minutes.

MUSCLE, WEAKNESS IN THE ELDERLY

HOME REMEDIES
- Yarrow tea: 2 cups daily.

MUSCULAR DYSTROPHY

VITAMINS / MINERALS
- A, B6, B12, E, C, B-complex, choline, inositol, pantothenic acid

MYOPIC ASTIGMATISM

HOME REMEDIES
- Tiger lily (*Lilium tigrinum*) (homeopathic)

NAILS

VITAMINS / MINERALS
- A, calcium, B2

NARCOTIC POISONING

HOME REMEDIES
- Bayberry tea or in capsules.

NAUSEA

HOME REMEDIES
- Summer savory: 1/2 tsp.
- Peach leaf tea (if constant)
- Flowers and oil of cloves.
- Nutmeg, peppermint, lemon balm, ginger, clove, and cinnamon also relieve nausea.

NEARSIGHTEDNESS

VITAMINS / MINERALS
- A, B-complex, C, E

NECK, ACHING

VITAMINS / MINERALS
- Magnesium

HOME REMEDIES
- Watch for reproductive organs out of harmony.

NECK, PAIN

HOME REMEDIES
- Comfrey root tea
- Rose petals
- Red clover tops
- Orange blossoms, nutmeg, mace

NEEDLES AND PINS

VITAMINS / MINERALS
- B12, folic acid

NEPHRITIS

VITAMINS / MINERALS
- A, B2, B6, choline, inositol, lecithin, calcium, magnesium, potassium, trace minerals from herb teas

HOME REMEDIES
- Watermelon seed tea

NEPHRITIS, ACUTE

HOME REMEDIES
- Elder flower tea: Drink 4 cups daily.

NERVE FOOD

VITAMINS / MINERALS
- Vitamin C

HOME REMEDIES
- Pineapple juice, prune juice: Combined, rebuilds exhausted nerves. Take 6 ozs. 3 times daily.
- Egg yolk: Two yolks from good healthy eggs mixed with 4 oz. grape juice once or twice daily.
- Apple whey: Take 1 pint apple juice or apple wine, 1 pint water, 1 pint milk. Heat it slowly but do not bring to a boil. When it curdles, strain it

through fine cloth. Throw curds away, sweeten with honey if needed. Take 2 tbls. 5 times daily if person is very weak. Appetite will improve and all signs of illness will disappear. As patient grows stronger, increase to 2 cups a day.
- Strawberries: Rich in vitamin C and minerals. Especially good for nervous disorders and to help build up weak kidney and bladder. Eat 4 ozs. 2 times daily.
- Cherry juice, egg yolk: Add egg yolk to a 6-ounce glass of cherry juice, stir, and drink.

NERVES (SEE ALSO SEDATIVES)

HOME REMEDIES
- Almonds: Blanch with grapes.
- Celery: Eat crisp and tender celery for depleted nerves.
- Sage: In bathtub and as tea.
- Lavender: In bathtub.
- Place a red and green towel in your bed. Sleep on it.
- St. John's wort oil: On painful spots.
- Lily, green leaves: Tie on painful spots.

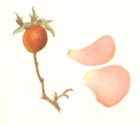

NERVES, IN KNOTS

HOME REMEDIES
- Lily oil

NERVES, INFLAMED/INFECTED (VERY PAINFUL)

HOME REMEDIES
- Peppermint tea
- Peppermint lotion: Applied locally

NERVES, INJURIES

HOME REMEDIES
- Daisy tea: 2 to 3 cups daily

NERVES, INVOLUNTARY NERVOUS SYSTEM

HOME REMEDIES
- Two-thirds of all nerve diseases are related to kidney trouble.
- Ginseng
- Horsetail tea

NERVES, PAIN IN ARMS AND LEGS

HOME REMEDIES
- Yarrow tea: 1 handful yarrow, brewed, strained, and added to bath.

NERVES, SEDATIVE

HOME REMEDIES
- Myrtle tea

NERVES, TONIC

HOME REMEDIES
- Oat water: Add to fruit juice.
- Barley water: Add to fruit juice.

NERVOUS, CONDITIONS

HOME REMEDIES
- Motherwort tea: 2 cups daily.
- Valerian root: 1/2 cup twice daily.
- Hops, St. John's wort, rosemary: Mix, make tea, and drink 2 cups daily.
- Caraway mixed with anise
- Bugleweed tea; Sage tea

NERVOUS DISORDERS

HOME REMEDIES
- Onion: Poultice to calves of legs does wonders.
- Marjoram
- Many nerve diseases have kidney trouble.

NERVOUS EXHAUSTION

HOME REMEDIES
- Silicon herbs

NERVOUS HEART PALPITATION

VITAMINS / MINERALS
- B-complex, B6, lecithin, magnesium, calcium, trace minerals from valerian root

HOME REMEDIES
- Rue tea (DO NOT take during pregnancy.)

NERVOUS SYSTEM, INVOLUNTARY

HOME REMEDIES
- Horsetail tea
- Ginseng

NERVOUS TENSION

HOME REMEDIES
- Catnip, mint: Make tea and drink 1 cup as needed.

NERVOUS WEAKNESS, AFTER ILLNESS

HOME REMEDIES
- Skullcap tea: 1/2 cup 3 times daily.

NERVOUSNESS

VITAMINS / MINERALS

- Magnesium, lecithin, calcium, B-complex, B6

HOME REMEDIES

- Mix hops, St. John's wort, and rosemary. Make a tea and drink 2 cups a day.

NEURALGIA

VITAMINS / MINERALS

- B-complex
- Allspice: Boil crushed fruit and apply on a cloth.

HOME REMEDIES

- St. John's wort (*Hypericum perforatum*) (homeopathic)
- Primrose
- Passion flowers: 2 cups daily.
- Salt: Heat in frying pan or oven. Put in a cloth bag and apply to painful face.
- White beet: Boil and apply to the pain in a small poultice sack.
- Mullein oil, yarrow oil, chamomile oil, thyme oil: Mix the oils and apply to pain.
- Chamomile tea
- Red onion: Use as a poultice.
- In ankle: Mullein
- In right ankle: Yarrow
- In lower jaw: Prickly ash; raw plantain juice over painful area.

NEURASTHENIA

HOME REMEDIES

- Gentian tea: Drink 1/2 cup twice daily.

NEURITIS, FROM ARSENIC POISON

VITAMINS / MINERALS

- B6, niacin

NEURITIS, FROM ALCOHOL, LEAD, DRUG POISON

VITAMINS / MINERALS

- B-complex, B6, niacin, trace minerals from okra, pumpkin

HOME REMEDIES

- Okra, pumpkin

NEURITIS, OF THE EYE

VITAMINS / MINERALS

- B-complex, B1

NEURITIS, IN LOWER EXTREMITIES

VITAMINS / MINERALS

- B6, niacin, B-complex

NEURITIS, UNKNOWN CAUSE

VITAMINS / MINERALS
- B-complex, B1, B15, B6, B12, lecithin, pantothenic acid, C-complex

HOME REMEDIES
- Combine avocado with agar-agar (dry), lime juice, and raw rolled oats. Drink plenty of distilled water between meals.

NIBBLING HABIT

HOME REMEDIES
- Alfalfa tablets
- Barberry tea: 1/2 cup 3 times daily.

NIGHT BLINDNESS

VITAMINS / MINERALS
- Vitamin A

HOME REMEDIES
- Club moss tea: 1 cup

NIGHT SWEATS, PROFUSE

HOME REMEDIES
- Dandelion leaf tea: 3 cups
- Linden blossom tea

NIGHTMARES

HOME REMEDIES
- Rosemary: A sprig under the pillow has been known to alleviate children's nightmares.

NOISE, DISTRACTION BY

VITAMINS / MINERALS
- B-complex, calcium, magnesium

HOME REMEDIES
- *Nux vomica* (homeopathic)

NOSE, BLEED

VITAMINS / MINERALS
- C, bioflavonoids, B15, B-complex, iron, K2 from alfalfa, trace minerals from okra

HOME REMEDIES
- Shepherd's purse: 2 cups daily.

NOSE, BLOWING FREQUENTLY

HOME REMEDIES
- Couch grass tea: 2 tbls. to 1 cup of water. Drink several cups daily.

NOSE, CHRONIC NASAL INFLAMMATION

HOME REMEDIES

- Bloodroot tea: $1/2$ cup 2 times daily.

NOSE, CRUSTS FORMING IN

VITAMINS / MINERALS

- Calcium fluoride

NOSE, DRY AND OBSTRUCTED

HOME REMEDIES

- Elder flower tea: 2 cups daily.
- Put arms in warm bath. Add sage to the water. Also boil basil in milk and steep a tsp. of sage in it. Drink 6 oz. a day. Sage boiled in milk, 2 tbls. several times a day.

NOSE, POLYPS

HOME REMEDIES

- A strong tea made of oak bark, sniffed up the nose several times daily.
- Dulcamara roots made in tea and sniffed several times a day.

NOSE, REDNESS

HOME REMEDIES

- Wash with a borax solution and rub strawberries over it.

NUMBNESS, IN FINGERTIPS AND TONGUE, LOWER LIP

HOME REMEDIES

- Chickpea (*Lathyrus sativus*) (homeopathic)
- Anise tea: For lower lip.

NURSING PAIN (GOES FROM NIPPLE ALL OVER BODY)

HOME REMEDIES

- Pokeroot tea: 2 cups daily.

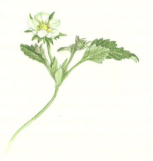

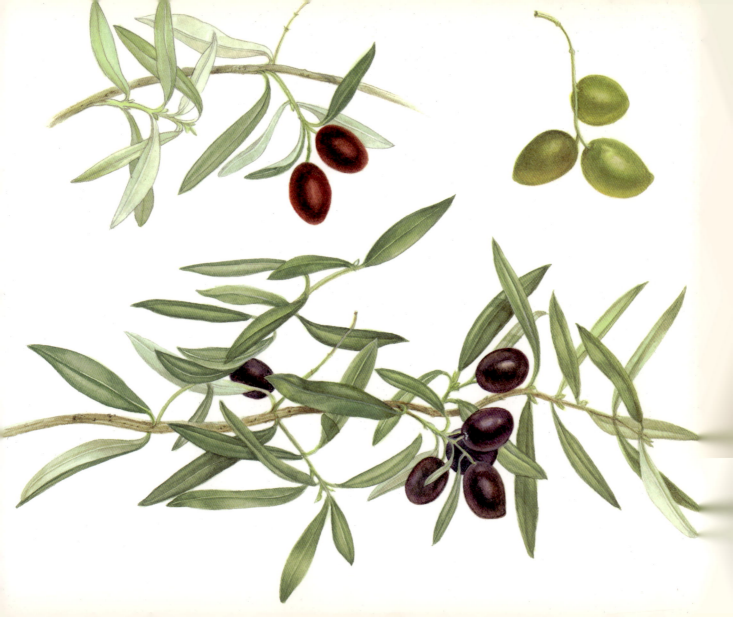

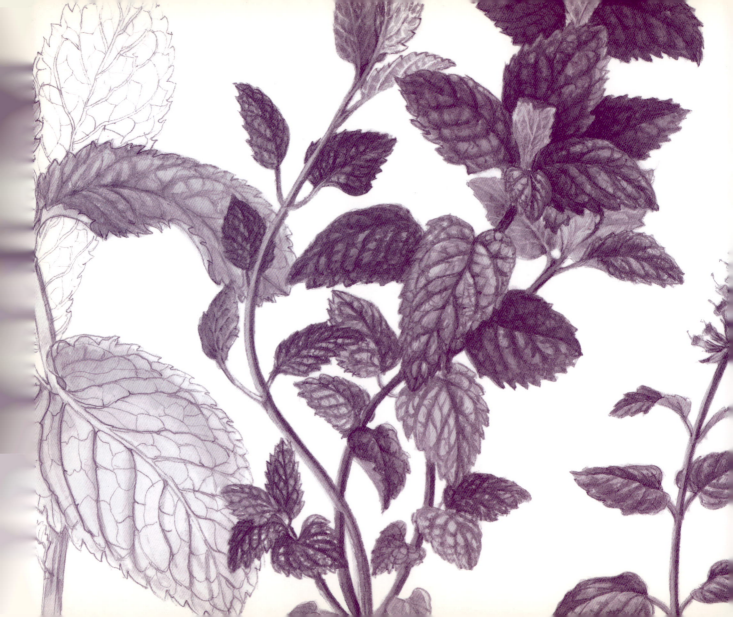

PAIN, BURNING

VITAMINS / MINERALS
- B12, folic acid

PAIN, FACIAL MUSCLE

VITAMINS / MINERALS
- B12, folic acid

PAIN, FINGERTIPS, HEAD, AND HEELS

VITAMINS / MINERALS
- Iron

HOME REMEDIES
- Alfalfa (releases pain in head and limbs)
- Blue Flag (homeopathic) (for head pain with nausea)
- Lady's slipper tea, lavender tea, lavender oil applied to temples (for nerve pain in head)
- St. John's wort (for pain in Achilles tendon)

PAIN, GENERAL

HOME REMEDIES
- Yams: For any kind of pain
- Lavender: In bags, applied hot, will quickly relieve almost any localized pain
- Echinacea: For pain of a wandering nature
- Pokeroot tea: For shifting pain

- Aconite (*Aconitum napellus*), comfrey (*Symphytum officinale*), chicory (*Chichorium intybus*), and English mandrake (*Tamus communis*)
- Strawberries: Contain organic salicylates (active ingredient in aspirin)
- Epsom salts: Pour 3 lbs. in bath and soak for 1/2 hour until pain recedes.
- Salt: Heat in a frying pan, put in cloth sack, and place on painful area; cover with hot water bottle.

PAIN, IN HANDS AND FEET

HOME REMEDIES
- Epsom salt: Put 1 tbl. in warm water; soak approx. 20 minutes.

PAIN, SHOULDER-ARM SYNDROME

VITAMINS / MINERALS
- Iron, copper, B12, folic acid

HOME REMEDIES
- Echinacea tea or in capsules: For pectoral muscles.

PALSY

HOME REMEDIES
- Onion: Eat 1 raw daily.

PANCREAS

VITAMINS / MINERALS

- Iodine: 1 drop in glass of water for trouble that can be detected by the sense of oppression in the stomach region

HOME REMEDIES

- Red beets
- Nutmeg: Use freshly ground and store it only briefly, for it becomes rancid easily and does not work. Take 1/2 tsp. in hot water to stimulate liver/pancreas.
- Calamus root: Chew the root.

PANCREAS, WEAK

HOME REMEDIES

- Blue flag (*Iris versicolor*) (homeopathic)

PANCREATITIS

HOME REMEDIES

- Blueberries and bananas

PARALYSIS, FACIAL MUSCLES

VITAMINS / MINERALS

- B12, folic acid

HOME REMEDIES

- Left side: Prickly ash tea—1 cup twice daily.

- Stroke: Tobacco water—Wash limbs with tobacco water.
- Tongue: Prickly ash—Chew herb.

PARASITES

HOME REMEDIES

- Garlic: Take 3 cloves of garlic and boil in 1 cup milk for 5 minutes. Cool and strain; drink every night for 10 nights in a row.
- Apple cider vinegar: Take 2 tsps. every day in 6 to 7 oz. water.
- Cloves, pumpkin, and pumpkin seeds also help rid body of worms/parasites.
- Lima bean pods and peach tree leaves alleviate microscopic parasites.
- For tapeworm: Take 5 parts juniper berries and 5 parts white oil for one day. (Pomegranate is also helpful.)
- Thyme: Used to treat roundworms, tapeworms, threadworms, and hookworms.

PARKINSON'S DISEASE

HOME REMEDIES

- Emu-mu (oil made from the emu bird and other special oils) removes blockage from the central nervous system in a short time.

PERSPIRATION

HOME REMEDIES

- To encourage: Drink Linden flower tea, hot lemonade.

PHLEBITIS (SEE ALSO VARICOSE VEINS)

VITAMINS / MINERALS

- C, E, bioflavonoids, trace minerals from white oak bark tea

HOME REMEDIES

- Witch hazel; Stone root (*Collinsonia canadensis*)
- Reduce salt; reduce meat.
- Black radish root, parsley leaves (herbal formula): 2 capsules every hour
- Goldenseal root capsule: 1 every hour
- Use cottage cheese compresses.
- White oak bark tea: 1 to 2 quarts

PILES, PAINFUL

VITAMINS / MINERALS

- Dates and milk instead of breakfast

HOME REMEDIES

- Silicon herbs, B6

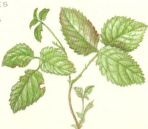

PIMPLES (SEE ALSO ACNE; BOILS AND PIMPLES)

HOME REMEDIES

- Lemon verbena tea: Dampen a clean cloth and scrub face vigorously. Repeat for 9 days and see an improvement.
- Epsom salts: Make a brine and pat on the face with cotton. Let dry before going to bed. Do this until pimples are dried up.

PINKEYE

HOME REMEDIES

- Potato: Raw, grated potatoes over closed eye. Or take thin slices of raw potato and cover eye. It will release pain, and the redness will go away. Red potatoes are best.
- Soak a clean cloth in warm water and apply to the eyes a few minutes several times a day. Be sure to wash anything that comes in contact with your eyes. See a doctor if it doesn't clear up in a few days.

PITUITARY, DEFICIENCY

HOME REMEDIES

- Cherry bark; cherry juice
- Alternate: 1 bunch of watercress one day, and 6 oz. pineapple juice 2 times the next day
- Wild cherry bark tincture: 7 drops twice daily

PLEURISY

HOME REMEDIES

- Flaxseed: As tea and as poultice
- Pleurisy root tea: Several cups
- Lady's mantle tea: 2 cups daily
- Thyme, fennel: Make tea. This combination relaxes.

PNEUMONIA

HOME REMEDIES

- Collard seeds, parsley seeds, spinach seeds, onion seeds: Simmer 1 tsp. of each of the seeds in 1 pint water. One pint water needs 4 tbls. of seeds. Drink 4 oz. every hour.
- Milk: Warm milk compresses around the upper torso. Take a towel, dip in warm milk, wrap around body. Wrap with plastic, then warm cloth.
- Also, hold right hand over forehead and left hand on lower back of head for 20 minutes.
- Cranberry juice: Preferred over any other juice

POISON IVY

HOME REMEDIES

- Epsom salts: Wet Epsom salts and apply to painful areas.
- Fels Naphtha soap: Wash with this soap—no more trouble.
- White oak bark tea bath; Sassafras tea bath; Tansy tea bath; *Rhus toxicodendron* (homeopathic)

POISON OAK

HOME REMEDIES

- White oak bark tea: Apply.
- Rub cream of tartar over the area.
- Homeopathic Anacardium is an antidote.

POISONS, FLUSHING FROM SYSTEM

HOME REMEDIES

- Combine anise and caraway: Make tea and drink 3 cups a day.

POISONS, SWALLOWED

HOME REMEDIES

- Charcoal: It will absorb up to $1/2$ its weight in poison. Burn a piece of bread, toasting it many times.

POLIOMYELITIS

HOME REMEDIES

- Chickpea (*Lathyrus sativus*) (homeopathic)

POLYPS

VITAMINS / MINERALS
- A, silicon

HOME REMEDIES
- For the mouth: Horsetail
- For the nose: Oak bark tea (strong). Sniff it into nose several times daily.

POTASSIUM, LACK OF

HOME REMEDIES
- Lady's mantle; banana

PREGNANCY

HOME REMEDIES
- Peaches: A complete food for mother and fetus. Also, drink peach leaf tea for morning sickness.
- Coconut milk: Pregnant women should take this regularly in the morning on an empty stomach. It will bring clear urine and also nourish the fetus. The child will be a healthy one.
- Ginger: Relieves morning sickness

PREMENSTRUAL SYNDROME (PMS)

VITAMINS / MINERALS
- Calcium, magnesium

HOME REMEDIES
- Cramp bark tea: 1 cup as needed
- Black cohosh
- Feed the adrenal glands.

PREMENSTRUAL TENSION

VITAMINS / MINERALS
- A

PROSTATE, ENLARGED

VITAMINS / MINERALS
- A, B-complex, C, E, F, potassium, trace minerals from fenugreek tea

HOME REMEDIES
- Couch grass
- Echinacea: 2 capsules 3 times daily
- Milk compresses: Make as you would give a diaper to a baby. Warm the milk (Do Not Boil), soak a Turkish or terry cloth towel (cotton) in it and apply as a diaper. Cover with a hot water bottle and place a plastic sheet underneath.

PROSTATE, GENERAL HEALTH

VITAMINS / MINERALS

- Zinc

HOME REMEDIES

- Coconut: Coconut milk is a specific for toning up the prostate gland.
- Myrrh: Cleanses the system
- Bee pollen; Pumpkin seed; Saw palmetto tincture

PROTEIN

HOME REMEDIES

- Avocado: Fat and protein supplier
- Lentils: Supply protein and iron of the best quality
- Meat: Gives explosive energy; appetite satisfying
- Millet: Vegetarian; 15 percent protein; millet is easily digested.

PSORIASIS

VITAMINS / MINERALS

- Iodine

HOME REMEDIES

- Celandine (*Chelidonium majus*) (homeopathic)
- Blue flag (*Iris versicolor*) (homeopathic)
- Nettle tea; Calendula tea
- Combine: Iodine (2 parts, not white), castor oil (4 parts). Mix and apply to skin once daily.
- Cool baths with apple cider vinegar added to water

PULSE (ALTERNATES OFTEN)

VITAMINS / MINERALS

- Iodine

PUS FORMATION

VITAMINS / MINERALS

- A, C, calcium, sulfur

HOME REMEDIES

- Vinegar: Take 2 tbls. vinegar, add to 1 quart water, heat, and inhale vapor for 10 minutes 3 or 4 times a day for pus formation of lungs, sinuses, and throat.

PYORRHEA

VITAMINS / MINERALS

- A, B-complex, B6, C, bioflavonoids, niacin, calcium, potassium

HOME REMEDIES

- Goldenseal, myrrh: Make tea and hold in mouth several times daily.
- Calamus root: Chew small pieces several times daily.
- Make your own toothpaste: Powdered calcium (bone meal is best), sage, myrrh and goldenseal (very little, for it is bitter).

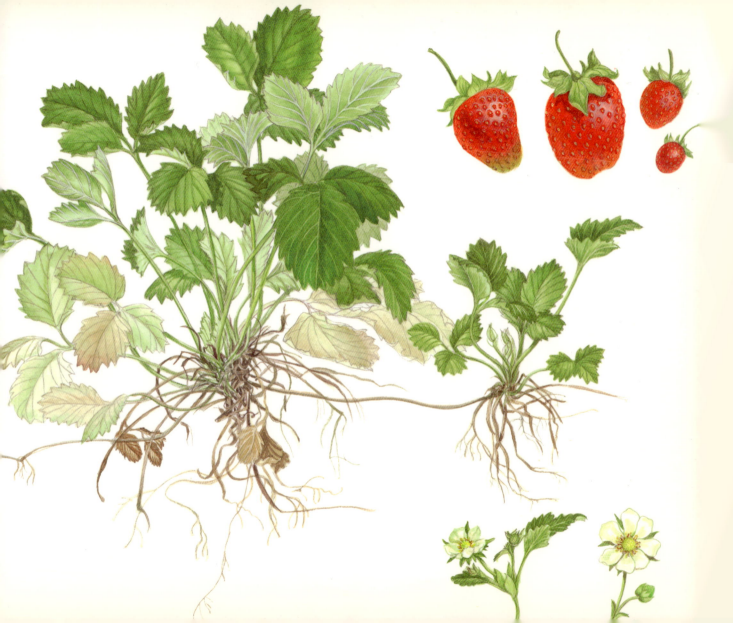

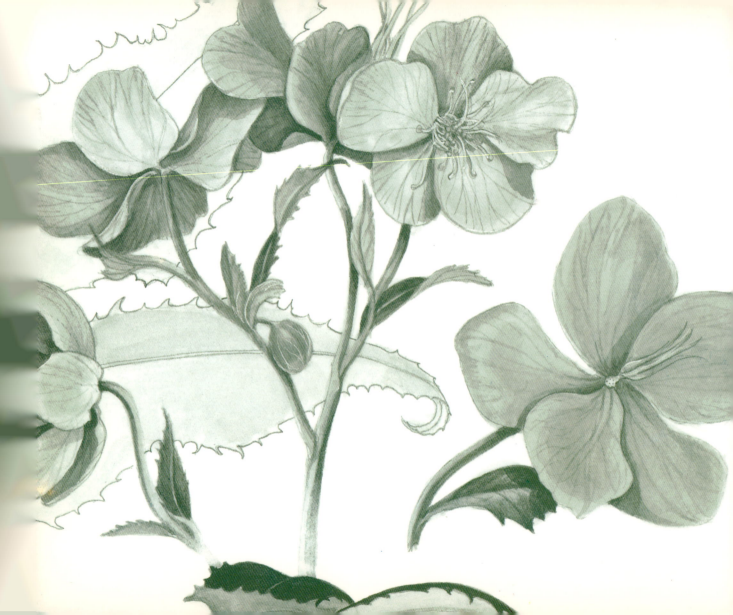

RADIATION

VITAMINS / MINERALS
- B6 (for side effects of)

HOME REMEDIES
- Clorox: Add 6 oz. of Clorox-brand bleach to your bath and soak for 10 to 15 minutes.
- Salt, baking soda: Add 1 pound of each to your bathwater and soak for 15 minutes.
- Seaweed: Has a neutralizing effect (so does Miso soup)

RECTUM, ACHING OR PROLAPSED

HOME REMEDIES
- Spikenard tea: 1/2 cup twice daily

RECTUM, ULCERATED

HOME REMEDIES
- Chlorophyll: Either in capsules or in liquid form

REPRODUCTIVE ORGANS, FEMALE (TO STRENGTHEN)

HOME REMEDIES
- Yarrow; Calendula; Nettle

REPRODUCTIVE ORGANS, INFECTION

HOME REMEDIES
- Oak bark concoction in bathtub

REPRODUCTIVE ORGANS, ITCHING OF GENITALS

HOME REMEDIES
- Wash with strong sage tea.

REPRODUCTIVE ORGANS, MALE (TO STRENGTHEN)

HOME REMEDIES
- Saw Palmetto (*Sabal serrulata*) (homeopathic)

RESISTANCE, LOW

HOME REMEDIES
- Calcium herbs

RESISTANCE TO DISEASE

HOME REMEDIES
- Thyme tea: Drink 1 cup daily.

RESPIRATORY AILMENTS

HOME REMEDIES

- Celery seed tea
- Hot lemon juice with honey can relieve cough and sore throats.
- Marjoram, violet leaves, chickweed are helpful.
- Thyme tea: 1 cup daily

RETINA, BLEEDING

VITAMINS / MINERALS

- C, bioflavonoids, rutin, B1

HOME REMEDIES

- Raw potato compresses
- Paprika (Hungarian is best): 1 tsp. on your food 3 times daily

RHEUMATIC FEVER

HOME REMEDIES

- Apple peeling concentrate

RHEUMATIC MUSCLES

HOME REMEDIES

- Asparagus
- Basil: Drink as tea and/or sprinkle on an oiled cloth and apply to ache.
- Sawdust: Contains natural DMSO. Take pine sawdust, boil in water for 10 minutes, and place hands or feet into the warm mush. When there is pain in the spine, strain the mush and place in sack and place on area.

RHEUMATISM

VITAMINS / MINERALS

- *Rumafix*, B-complex, B, B15, C, bioflavonoids, folic acid, calcium (in many cases, but not all)

HOME REMEDIES

- Chickweed: If shifting from side to side.
- Violet root: In upper part of body, right side.
- Basil: Drink as tea and/or sprinkle on an oiled cloth and apply to ache.
- Raw potato: Carry a raw potato in your pocket. In 1 or 2 days, it's shriveled up and smells from the poison attracted. Replace it with another potato.
- Marjoram tea or oil in bathwater. Or put a drop of oil on the pillow to induce sleep.
- Oregano: Apply externally.
- Oil extracted from borage seeds: Available in capsules
- Avocado: Combine with Agar-agar (dry), lime juice, and raw rolled oats. Drink plenty of distilled water between meals.
- Horsetail tea or in capsules for pain
- Rosemary: Stimulates circulation and eases pain

RHINITIS, CHRONIC (NASAL INFLAMMATION)

HOME REMEDIES
- Bloodroot tea: ½ cup twice daily

RICKETS

VITAMINS / MINERALS
- D, C, calcium, kelp baths

RINGWORM (TINEA)

HOME REMEDIES
- Banana peel: Rub peel on area.
- Bloodroot: Externally apply strong tea. Also, peel and rub on area.

ROSACEA

VITAMINS / MINERALS
- B12 (red nose)

SALIVA, PROFUSE FLOW

VITAMINS / MINERALS
- Calcium (for too much in throat)
HOME REMEDIES
- Plantain
- Blue flag (*Iris versicolor*) (homeopathic)

SALIVA, TO INCREASE

HOME REMEDIES
- Prickly ash tea
- Sage: Chew leaves
- Cloves: Chew

SCABIES

HOME REMEDIES
- Thyme tea: Use as a skin antiseptic.

SCARS

VITAMINS / MINERALS
- Calcium
- Vitamin E taken externally and applied to scars
HOME REMEDIES
- Peppermint oil: Rub on scar.
- Cocoa butter: Rub on scar. It has to be done consistently, twice daily.
- Homeopathic: *Drosera rotundifolia;* a remedy specific for graphites

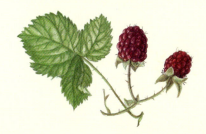

SCIATICA

VITAMINS / MINERALS

- B-complex, B1, B15

HOME REMEDIES

- Pinkroot, St. John's wort, cayenne pepper, black tea: Mix and drink 1 cup.
- Elderberry juice: Specific for sciatica
- Elderberry tea: Also good
- Mugwort: If sciatica is worse in hot weather, use this.
- Fenugreek: Make poultice of hot milk and crushed seeds.

SCURVY

VITAMINS / MINERALS

- C, bioflavonoids

HOME REMEDIES

- Increase green leafy vegetables and fruit intake.
- Dog rose (*Rosa canina*)

SEASICKNESS

HOME REMEDIES

- Pennyroyal: Carry it with you when traveling.

SEBORRHEA, ON FACE, LIPS, AND MOUTH

VITAMINS / MINERALS

- B6

SEBORRHEIC DERMATITIS

VITAMINS / MINERALS

- A, B-complex, biotin

SHINGLES

VITAMINS / MINERALS

- B-complex, B1, B12, folic acid

HOME REMEDIES

- Peppermint tea: Use as an eyewash or skin wash.
- Celery: 1 1/2 quarts celery juice daily
- Epsom salts: Make a paste by adding water to achieve the right consistency, then apply frequently to the affected parts until relief is felt.
- Take 4 oz. witch hazel or spirit of camphor, add 8 drops of peppermint oil, shake, and apply to painful area.
- Leeks: Blend some of the leaves in the blender with a little water and apply to the painful area.
- *Arsenicum metallicum; Ranunculus bulbosus* (homeopathic)

SHOCK

HOME REMEDIES

- Cayenne pepper in cream
- Eating oranges calms the nerves.
- Hypericum or St. John's wort

SHOULDER, ARM SYNDROME (PAIN)

VITAMINS / MINERALS

- Iron, copper, B1, folic acid

SHOULDER, PAIN

HOME REMEDIES

- Under right shoulder: Gallbladder
- Under left shoulder: Stomach

SHOULDER, RIGHT (PAIN/ STIFFNESS TO RAISE ARM)

HOME REMEDIES

- Pokeroot tea: 2 cups daily

SINUS

VITAMINS / MINERALS

- A, C, bioflavonoids

HOME REMEDIES

- Horseradish, onion, turnips, mustard, radishes

- Horseradish: Take a piece of fresh horseradish, or open a jar of horseradish relish and take a little piece several times a day.
- Black pepper: Take 1 tsp. honey, grind black pepper over it (it must be freshly ground), and take as needed.
- Add 1 tbl. marjoram to one tbl. butter, boil 5 minutes and strain through cloth. Rub forehead, nose, cheeks, and nostrils with it.
- Sip 12 ozs. grape juice twice daily for 6 weeks.
- Garlic: Nature's antibiotic; will help fight infection

SKIN

HOME REMEDIES

- Comfrey: Combine with any good face or hand lotion to produce a product that has been found valuable in removing various imperfections on the skin and, in some instances, will cause wrinkles to disappear.
- Cucumbers: Either eat or apply topically. They cool and heal the skin.

SKIN, AILMENTS

HOME REMEDIES

- Slippery elm: Make a poultice for skin ailments such as burns, boils, and ulcers.

- *Thuja occidentalis*, staph, or *Arsenicum* (homeo-pathic)

SKIN, BLEMISHES

HOME REMEDIES

- Combine 1/3 tsp. ground nutmeg, 1 tsp. honey, and 4 to 5 oz. hot water; take 3 mornings in a row, then a 3-day break; repeat 9 times.
- Garlic: Rub fresh garlic cloves on skin.
- Soda bicarbonate: Make a small paste of spirits of camphor in soda bicarbonate, pat on area, and leave on overnight for 1 week. Do not bandage or cover for 1 week.

SKIN, BLOOD PURIFIER

HOME REMEDIES

- Strawberry leaves; Primrose (*Primula officinalis*); Nettle;
- Ground ivy

SKIN, DRY AND CHAPPED

HOME REMEDIES

- Cocoa butter (part), glycerin (1 part), lanolin (1 part), rose water (1 part), elder flower water (1 part): Mix and apply to skin daily.
- Mix 3 drops lemon oil and 3 drops glycerin: Apply to chapped hands and skin.

SKIN, ECZEMA

HOME REMEDIES

- Strawberry leaf tea
- Club moss behind the ear
- Pansy tea (for children)
- Evening primrose oil on joints and fingers

SKIN, INFECTION

HOME REMEDIES

- White pond lily: Apply to skin.

SKIN, PIGMENTATION (DIRTY, OILY, YELLOWISH)

VITAMINS / MINERALS

- Calcium fluoride

SKIN, RED AND SCALY

VITAMINS / MINERALS

- A, B2, lecithin

HOME REMEDIES

- Soybean lecithin for red, itchy, scaly skin. Make a salve and apply. Also take 2 tbls.

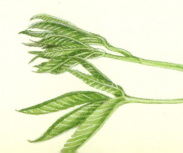

SKIN, REMEDIES

HOME REMEDIES

- Cucumber: Contains a hormone needed by the pancreas to produce insulin. It is specific for skin trouble.
- Coconut oil: Massage on scalp and all over body in summer. Applied with success on eczema, dermatitis, etc.
- Myrrh: Found to help athlete's foot, eczema, cracked skin, ringworm, and wrinkles

SKIN, TUMORLIKE ERUPTIONS

HOME REMEDIES

- Sheep sorrel: Wash skin with strong tea.

SKUNK ODOR

HOME REMEDIES

- Tomato juice: Wash body and clothes with $^{1}/_{2}$ cup tomato juice in water and/or $^{1}/_{2}$ cup ammonia in water.

SLEEPLESSNESS

VITAMINS / MINERALS

- B1, iron (for sleeplessness at night and sleepy during the day)

HOME REMEDIES

- Dill seeds: Simmer in olive oil and rub on forehead.
- Cowslip: Sweetened with honey
- Poppy seed: Fill a small sock and lay it on your forehead.
- Laurel leaves: Place in a small bag and lay your head on it.
- Anise seed: Take 1 tsp. before going to bed.
- Honey and milk: Warm a cup of milk, add 1 tsp. of honey, and drink before going to bed.
- Foot bath: At night, take a hot foot bath so poisons are eliminated. Rub soles of feet with a slice of lemon after foot bath.
- Chamomile tea; lemon balm tea; alfalfa
- Nutmeg tea: Use sparingly because large doses can be poisonous and can cause miscarriage.

SLEEPWALKING

HOME REMEDIES

- Mugwort tea

SMOKING HABIT

HOME REMEDIES

- Calamus root: Found to rebuild the lungs from smoking damage. Combine 1 rounded tsp. calamus root and 1 qt. apple juice. Boil for 15 minutes, strain, and drink 6 oz., 3 times daily.

STAPH INFECTION

HOME REMEDIES

- Savory: Antibacterial, antifungal, and antiviral
- Oxoquiniline: From the quinine tree
- A specific homeopathic remedy for staph

STERILITY

VITAMINS / MINERALS

- A, B-complex, E

STOMACH

HOME REMEDIES

- Healing to sick stomachs, ulcers, and pain: Carrot, coconut milk, eggplant, flaxseed tea, okra, parsnip, sweet potato.
- Indian remedy: Blackberry wine
- Ironweed, cashew (*Anacardium occidentale*), cleavers
- Calamus root: uncooked
- Unsweetened pineapple juice poured over melons develops pepsin, which is needed for digestion.
- Persimmon: Take before meals if stomach does not behave.
- Cardamom: Has a soothing effect on all membranes of the stomach and lungs
- Whey: Take 1 tbl. 3 times daily. This will feed the stomach glands, and they will work well again.

STOMACH, ACHE

HOME REMEDIES

- Flaxseed: Take 2 tsps., cover with 8 ozs. boiling water, keep it warm for 30 minutes, and drink 1 to 2 cups.

STOMACH, CRAMPS

HOME REMEDIES

- Apricot brandy: This will stop chronic stomach cramps. Take 1 tsp.

STOMACH, FLU

HOME REMEDIES

- Ginger: Use 1/2 tsp. ground ginger to 1 cup water. Add 1 tsp. honey and drink hot. Also, hot compresses of ginger over stomach will bring relief.

STOMACH, GAS

HOME REMEDIES

- Certo, apple juice: 1 tsp. Certo added to 1/2 glass apple juice, drink as needed

STOMACH, HEAVINESS

HOME REMEDIES

- Ginger tea or Violet leaf tea

STOMACH, SOUR

HOME REMEDIES
- Raw potato slices: Eat.
- Charcoal tablets

STOMACH, ULCERS

VITAMINS / MINERALS
- A from carrots—carotene; B from rice polishings, E, C, bioflavonoids, K2, aloe vera juice for trace minerals

HOME REMEDIES
- Marigold tea, yarrow tea
- Cabbage: Cabbage juice (it must be freshly made) is used for stomach ulcers because of vitamin U in cabbage.
- Okra: Cooked, do not season heavily
- Potato: Juice 1 potato, add the same amount of warm water. Drink before each meal, 3 times a day. Red potatoes are best.
- Apples: Raw and cooked
- Calamus root tea: Cut root and let stand overnight in water. Then warm it (do not boil). Sip 1/2 cup before meals.

STOMACH, UPSET

HOME REMEDIES
- Cinnamon: Drink or chew on sticks.

- Pumpkin: High in beta carotene and calms upset stomach

STOMACH, WEAK

HOME REMEDIES
- Gentian: Use very little.
- Powdered okra; slippery elm tea; rosemary

STOOL, CLAY COLORED

HOME REMEDIES
- Chickweed
- Goldenrod, goldenseal root, cloves (herbal formula)

STREP INFECTION

HOME REMEDIES
- Cucumber: Grate and squeeze the juice out. Drink 5 times a day.
- Chinese sumach (*Ailanthus Glandulosa*) (homeopathic)

STRESS

VITAMINS / MINERALS
- A, B-complex, B12, folic acid, C, E, calcium, D, phosphorus, pantothenic acid

STRETCH MARKS

VITAMINS / MINERALS
- Vitamin E ointment

STROKE

VITAMINS / MINERALS
- C, bioflavonoids, E, choline, potassium

HOME REMEDIES
- Lavender tea: Drink 2 cups.
- Angelica root tea: Drink 1 cup.
- Mustard seed: Every morning thoroughly chew 1 tsp.
- Tofu: Shave head, apply tofu over head, and change the compress when tofu gets yellow.

STROKE, PARALYSIS AFTER

HOME REMEDIES
- Wash the limbs with tobacco water.

STY

HOME REMEDIES
- Eyebright (*Euphrasia officinalis*) (homeopathic)
- Castor oil
- Burdock root tea: Drink it and apply.
- Black tea (Lipton will do): Make a poultice, place moist over the eye, bandage at night.

SUNBURN

VITAMINS / MINERALS
- A, calcium without D, PABA ointment

HOME REMEDIES
- Aloe vera
- Cornstarch: Mix with water to make a paste and apply to sunburn. Will ease pain.
- Lettuce leaves: Boil, strain, and let the liquid cool several hours in the refrigerator. Apply gently to sunburn.

SWELLING

HOME REMEDIES
- Lettuce water: Apply externally over swollen parts of body.
- Raw cabbage poultice: Grate into a cheesecloth and apply overnight. Use several nights in a row for best results.
- Tomato: A slice on swelling reduces it quickly.
- Adzuki beans: Boil in plenty of water. Eat them as a soup, or drink the fluid twice daily.

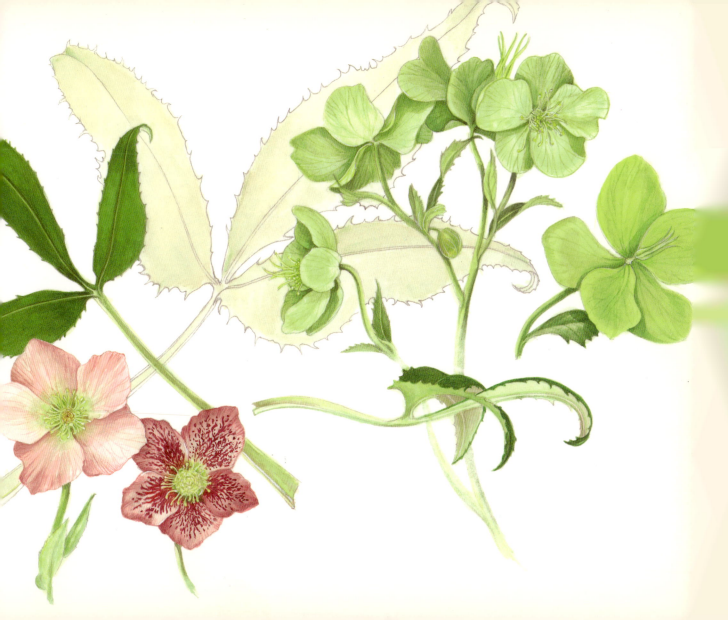

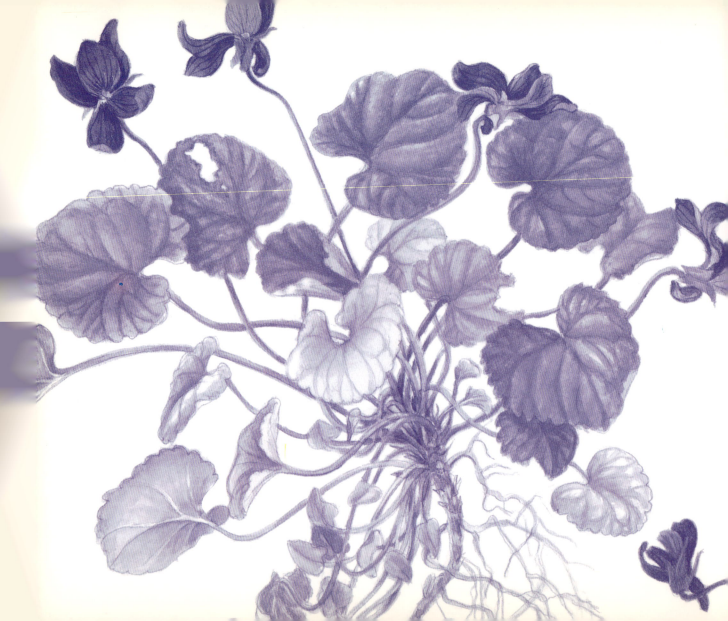

TACHYCARDIA

HOME REMEDIES

- Hawthorn, blessed thistle, red roses: Mix equal parts, make tea, and drink 2 cups daily.

TAPEWORM

HOME REMEDIES

- Pomegranate twigs: Boil and drink 3 cups daily during the full moon for 3 days in a row.

TEETH, CLENCHED

HOME REMEDIES

- Pokeroot tea: Drink 1 cup three times daily.

TENSION

HOME REMEDIES

- Carrot seeds: Make a tea and drink a cup now and then. It will remove tension from the smooth muscles such as the intestines.

TESTICLES, SWOLLEN

VITAMINS / MINERALS

- Potassium, trace minerals from fenugreek
- Echinacea: In capsule form

THROAT, DRY

VITAMINS / MINERALS

- B2

THROAT, LUMP IN (GLOBUS HYSTERICUS)

HOME REMEDIES

- St. Ignatius' bean (*Ignatia amara*) (homeopathic)
- Blue malva: Let sit overnight in cold water.

THROAT, SORE

HOME REMEDIES

- Sage tea: Gargle:
- Arnica tincture: Use 2 to 3 drops in 1 tbl. of warm water.
- Sea salt in vinegar water: Gargle.

THROMBOSIS

VITAMINS / MINERALS

- C, bioflavonoids, rutin, trace minerals from white oak bark

HOME REMEDIES

- White oak bark tea

THYMUS, SECRETION INSUFFICIENT

HOME REMEDIES
- Copper herbs

THYROID, ENLARGED

HOME REMEDIES
- Pokeroot compresses: Apply overnight.

THYROID, SLUGGISH

VITAMINS / MINERALS
- A, B-complex, C, E, choline, iodine, trace minerals from kelp (for underactive condition)

HOME REMEDIES
- Kelp or seaweed

TOBACCO, CRAVING

HOME REMEDIES
- Laurel leaves: Make a tea and also put in soups or meat dishes.

TONGUE, BURNING

HOME REMEDIES
- Blue Malva Tea: Boil and hold 1 tsp. in mouth.

TONGUE, FISSURES

VITAMINS / MINERALS
- B2

HOME REMEDIES
- Raspberry leaf tea: Hold in mouth several times a day.

TONGUE, SORES

HOME REMEDIES
- Raspberry leaf tea: Hold in mouth several times daily.

TONSILS, SWOLLEN

HOME REMEDIES
- Banana: Baked in the skin and mashed with a little fresh cream or olive oil. Make compresses. Don't eat bananas for cold or cough; they will add to the problems.
- Grapefruit juice
- Savory tea: Use as an antiseptic mouthwash and gargle.

TOOTHACHE

VITAMINS / MINERALS
- Magnesium (for ache when nothing is wrong)

HOME REMEDIES

- Black tea: Soak a black tea bag in hot water, apply to cheek.
- Hyssop: Between tooth and gum overnight
- Cloves: A little clove oil inserted into the cavity Powdered milk in the hole will stop the ache for a while, also.
- Pepper and mustard: Place on a piece of cloth and put over aching cheek.
- Oregano: Chewing on the leaf provides temporary relief.
- Cayenne: Rub on toothache.

TOOTH, BLEEDING AFTER EXTRACTION

HOME REMEDIES

- Black tea: After extraction, take one Lipton black tea bag, wet it in warm water, and apply.

TOOTH, DECAY

HOME REMEDIES

- Boil 1 cup of chopped mulberry bark or fine twigs in 1 quart concord grape juice for $1/2$ hour. Take 1 tbl. 6 times daily. Keep it in your mouth, then swallow.
- Citrus fruits, licorice root extract, soy products, and curcumin prevent dental decay.
- Cheese: Eat aged cheese, such as cheddar, to prevent the formation of plaque.

TOOTH, LOOSE

HOME REMEDIES

- Apple cider vinegar: Hold warm apple cider vinegar in your mouth, spit it out. Do this several times a day.
- Sage: Boil with honey and hold in mouth.

TOOTH, POWDER

HOME REMEDIES

- Soda and salt

TOOTH, STRENGTHENER

HOME REMEDIES

- Bonemeal

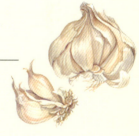

TOXICITY

VITAMINS / MINERALS

- Sulfur

TRENCH MOUTH

HOME REMEDIES

- Raspberry, oak bark: Make a juice and spray it in mouth.

TRICHINOSIS

HOME REMEDIES

- Oil of wintergreen

TRIGLYCERIDES, ELEVATED

HOME REMEDIES

- Can be a sign of diabetes or liver problems. High risk factor in cardiovascular disease and stroke. To treat: Do moderate exercise, avoid sugar, eat high-fiber diet, eliminate red meat.

TUMOR

HOME REMEDIES

- Eggplant peelings: Boil and take 2 tbls. 2 times daily.
- Tomatoes: (including juice) Contain lycopene, which is known to reduce tumors. Apply raw tomatoes to head in case of brain tumors.
- Turmeric: Use a small amount to halt tumor growth.
- Turnips: Used for deep-rooted tumors; also, deep-rooted resentments
- Flax oil: Use for simple tumors.

TUMOR, FATTY

HOME REMEDIES

- Asparagus: Canned—the cheap ones are best. Blend it and take 2 tbls. in the morning and at night. Put it on bread or eat it alone.

- Bible remedy: Take 1 pound white figs in 3 quarts milk, boil until well done. Place figs in a blender, make a poultice, and apply overnight. Renew this every 12 hours for 3 days. Also, drink cup of this fig milk 3 times daily.

TUMOR, FIBROID

HOME REMEDIES

- Goldenrod tea
- Calendula (2 parts), yarrow (1 part), nettle (1 part): Mix and drink 1 quart daily for 4 weeks.

TUMOR, ILL-NATURED (LIVER)

HOME REMEDIES

- Calamus root: 1/2 cup 2 times daily.
- Goldenrod, goldenseal root, cloves (herbal formula)

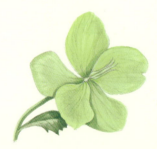

ULCERS

- B-complex, B12, folic acid, C, E, iron, K2 from alfalfa

HOME REMEDIES

- Calendula tea
- Calamus root: Chew:
- Ginger: About $1/4$ tsp. to 6 oz. hot water relieves upset stomach

ULCERS, DUODENAL

HOME REMEDIES

- Calamus root: Let sit in cold water: overnight. Warm it in the morning (do not boil). Drink cup 4 to 5 times daily.
- Comfrey root tea: 2 cups daily
- 12-herb tincture formula*
- Red potatoes

ULCERS, MOUTH

HOME REMEDIES

- Sage or willow leaves
- Blackberry leaf tea: Hold in mouth.

ULCERS, PEPTIC (GASTRIC)

VITAMINS / MINERALS

- Vitamin U deficiency

HOME REMEDIES

- Thought to be cased by stress and/or dyspepsia. Treatment should include alfalfa, cabbage juice, flax, German chamomile, and licorice.
- Consult physician.

ULCERS, STOMACH

HOME REMEDIES

- Calamus root tea: Cut root and let stand overnight in water. Then warm it (Do Not Boil). Sip $1/2$ cup before meals.
- Marigold tea; Yarrow tea; Nettle tea; Blue Malva Tea
- Carrots: Cooked, relieve stomach ulcers.
- Fenugreek relieves ulcer of the stomach.
- Red potatoes

UREA, EXCESSIVE

HOME REMEDIES

- Senna leaf tea; Juniper berry tea; Horsetail grass tea
- See a physician about magnesium deficiency.

UREMIA

HOME REMEDIES

- Epsom salts drink: 1 tsp. Epsom salts in 7 ozs. water every hour for 4 hours.

For more information, see page iii.

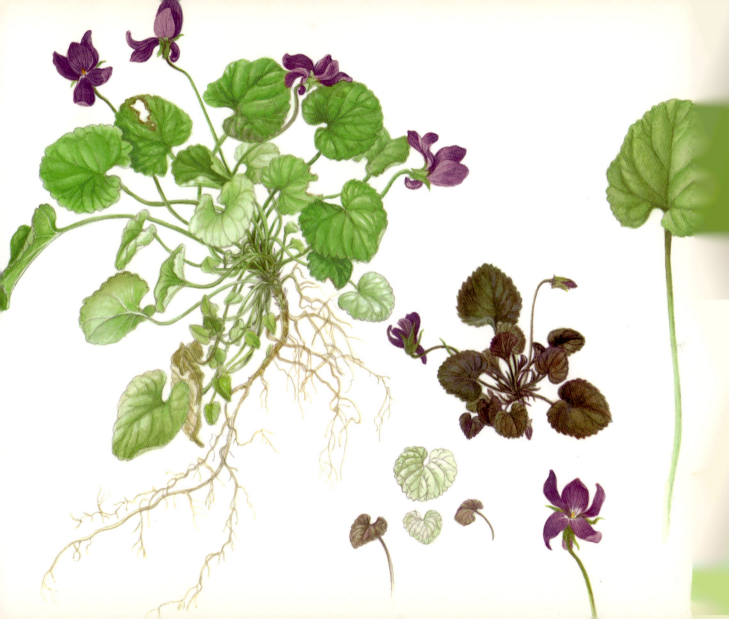

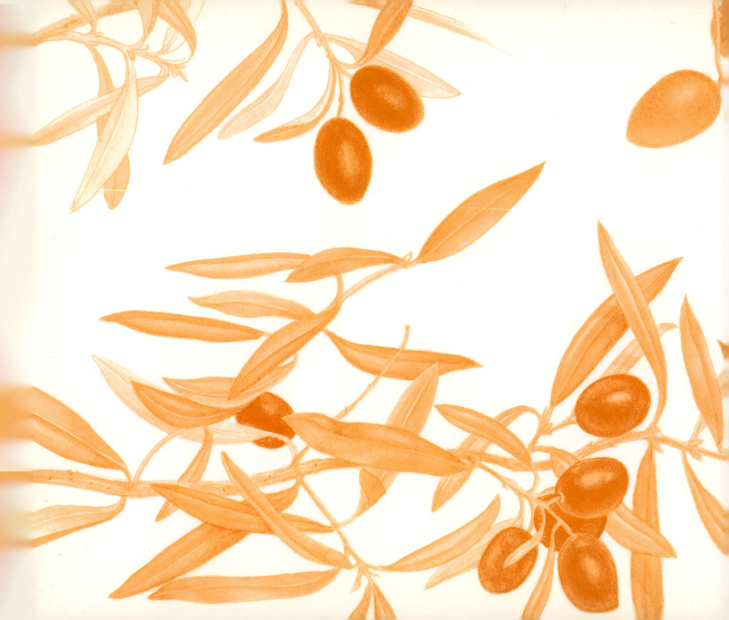

VAGINAL DISCHARGE

VITAMINS / MINERALS
- A, B-complex, B2, B6, C, E, iron, trace minerals

VARICOSE VEINS

VITAMINS / MINERALS
- Need zinc supplements

HOME REMEDIES
- Marigold: 1 oz. powdered flowers and stems with 1 pint of boiling water, allow to cool and apply directly to various affected parts of the body (for varicose veins, chronic ulcers, and similar ailments).
- Oak bark tea compress: Apply overnight.
- Plantain, yarrow, mullein, calendula: Mix, make tea, and drink 3 cups daily.
- Calendula salve: Apply.
- Cottage cheese compress: If possible, all night or just for several hours. Do this every night until gone.
- Cabbage: Grate and fill a piece of cheesecloth. Tie over painful areas and let sit overnight. (Do the same with head lettuce.)
- Sage: Apply hot compresses to legs. Take frequent sage foot baths.
- Homeopathic: *Arsenicum album*; Horse chestnut *(Aesculus hippocastanum)*; St. Mary's thistle *(Carduus marianus)*

VARICOSE VEINS, PREGNANCY

HOME REMEDIES
- Daisy tea

VARICOSE VEINS, PURPLE

HOME REMEDIES
- Horse chestnut

VASCULAR CONGESTION

HOME REMEDIES
- Whey: The transparent liquid released when yogurt or cheese is made. Whey removes vascular congestion and is a mind booster.

VERTIGO

HOME REMEDIES
- Crab apples: Boil and eat 1 tsp. every hour.
- Violet leaves
- Daisy tea (in elderly)

VIRAL INFECTION

VITAMINS / MINERALS
- C, bioflavonoids, A, trace minerals from sweet basil and lettuce water

HOME REMEDIES
- Calendula tea

- Cinnamon, chickpeas, lettuce, basil, romaine
- Lettuce water: Take leaf lettuce and boil in water, drink 4 ozs. every hour.
- Echinacea (homeopathic): For viral infections in blood and lymph

VISION, DIMNESS

HOME REMEDIES

- Linden flower, carrot juice, kidney tea

VITALITY, LOW

VITAMINS / MINERALS

- B-complex, B1, C, E, pantothenic acid

VITAMIN C REPLACEMENT

HOME REMEDIES

- Alfalfa seed
- Cranberry juice: Frequently recommended for people whose body is not utilizing vitamin C properly. The best time to drink it is early afternoon. Make sure you drink cranberry juice and not cranapple or other mixes.

VOMITING OF FOOD (CHRONIC)

HOME REMEDIES

- Vinegar: In case of severe vomiting, moisten a cloth with warm vinegar and apply over abdomen.
- Dill seed: Use 1/2 tsp. in water or chew it.
- Cinnamon and nutmeg also help relieve nausea.

WARTS

VITAMINS / MINERALS

- A, E, silicon

HOME REMEDIES

- Fenugreek seed: Soak seed in water until it makes a mucilage-like ointment. Apply to the wart and let dry. Use once daily until the wart disappears.
- Castor oil: Apply a few drops to wart and bandage tightly. Repeat 2 or 3 times daily until wart disappears.
- Dandelion juice or milkweed juice: Apply topically.
- Lemon peel: For calluses, corns, or warts. Put the lemon peel (white side down) on the afflicted area overnight.
- *Thuja occidentalis* (homeopathic)
- Dulcamara (homeopathic): Use for warts on hands and face.
- Willow leaf (fresh): Squeeze the juice on the wart.

WARTS, PLANTAR (FOOT)

HOME REMEDIES

- Chalk: Oil a piece of cloth, grate regular chalk over the oiled area and apply overnight. Do this for 14 days.

WATER RETENTION

VITAMINS / MINERALS

- Potassium

HOME REMEDIES

- Banana is a good potassium fruit. If taken in moderation, will balance excess water in the system.
- Fennel, watermelon seed tea, parsley tea
- Nettle (2 parts), uva ursi (1 part): Mix, make tea, and drink 4 cups daily to eliminate excess water from the cells.
- Woodruff tea: 3 cups daily

WEAKNESS, IN THE ELDERLY AND DEBILITATED

HOME REMEDIES

- Yarrow tea: Drink 2 cups daily.
- Arrowroot: It is easily digested, creating no gastric upset.

WEIGHT LOSS (SEE ANTIFAT, OBESITY, OVERWEIGHT)

WHOOPING COUGH

VITAMINS / MINERALS

- B6

HOME REMEDIES

- Red clover
- Also, rub onion juice into soles of feet or into the back. Or ginger tea or 1 tbl. thyme, boil in 1 cup water for 20 minutes, strain, add honey, take 1 tsp. every hour.

WORMS

VITAMINS / MINERALS

- Calcium (when worms are repeated)

HOME REMEDIES

- White figs are useful for de-worming. Figs and fig juice paralyze any worm, even the tapeworm, pinworm, and roundworm.
- Birch leaves or bark; Blue cohosh
- Garlic: Cut 3 cloves, boil in 8 ozs. of milk for 5 minutes, let cool so you can drink it. Do this before going to sleep for 10 days in a row.
- Pomegranate: As juice or eaten raw. Helps keep worms out of system.

- Pumpkin seeds: Eat ¹/₂ cup pumpkin seeds a day, especially before a meal on an empty stomach. Worms are stripped from their protective skins by pumpkin seeds.
- Figs: Eat 3 or 4 figs twice daily.

WRINKLES

HOME REMEDIES
- Cowslip oil
- Hellebore: for forehead
- Violet root: for hands and feet
- White hellebore tea: Wash in it; also for hands and feet.

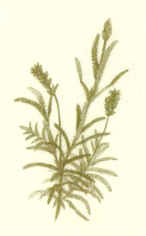

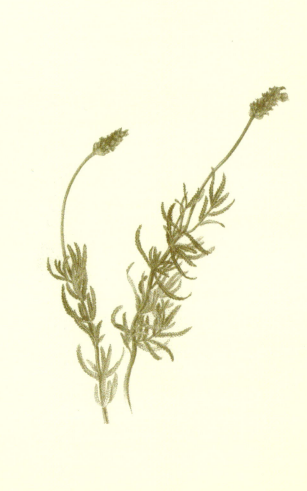

HERBS AND FORMULAS

Any herb types referred to in previous chart are included here. The herbs are categorized for your convenience, and healing oil and tincture recipes are also included.

CATEGORIZING HERBS

We are accustomed to categorizing our lives and also our environments. Reluctantly, I do so with herbs—the medicine of the ages, the medicine of God's drugstore.

This outline is only a small portion of herbs in your vicinity. By walking through the meadows, you will easily find the iron herbs, the magnesium herbs, and so on.

CALCIUM HERBS

Caraway seeds, Chamomile, Chives, Cleavers, Coltsfoot, Dandelion, Dill, Horsetail, Pimpernel, Tormentil root

CHLORINE HERBS

Fennel, Goldenseal, Myrrh, Nettle, Plantain, Uva Ursi, Watercress, Wintergreen

COPPER HERBS

Dandelion, Devil's Bit, Liverwort, Salep, Sheep Sorrel

FLUORINE HERBS

Cornsilk, Dill, Horsetail, Oats, Plantain, Thyme, Watercress

IODINE HERBS

Algae, Dulse, Iceland Moss, Irish Moss, Kelp, Mustard, Nettle, Parsley, Sea Wrack

IRON HERBS

Burdock, Dandelion, Huckleberry Leaves, Irish Moss, Meadowsweet, Sheep Sorrel, Silverweed, Stinging Nettle, Strawberry Leaves, Yellow Dock

MAGNESIUM HERBS

Broom Tops, Carrot Leaves, Devil's Bit, Meadowsweet, Mullein Leaves, Nettle, Primrose, Walnut Leaves

MANGANESE HERBS

Burdock, Kelp, Sheep Sorrel, Strawberry Leaves, Wintergreen, Yellow Dock

NICKEL HERBS

Algae, Bladderwrack, Kelp, Liverwort

POTASSIUM HERBS

American Centaury, Carrot Leaves, Comfrey, Couch Grass, Mullein, Oak Bark, Plantain Leaves, Primrose Flowers, Summer Savory, Walnut Leaves, Yarrow

PHOSPHORUS HERBS

Calamus, Chickweed, Dill, Licorice Root, Marigold Flowers, Rhubarb, Sorrel, Watercress

SILICON HERBS

Chickweed, Cornsilk, Flaxseed, Horsetail, Lamb's-quarters, Oat Straw, Red Raspberry Leaves, Sunflower Seeds

SODIUM HERBS

Apple Tree Bark, Celery Seed, Cleavers, Dill, Fennel Seed, Huckleberry Leaves, Meadowsweet, Mistletoe, Stinging Nettle

SULFUR HERBS

Coltsfoot, Eyebright, Fennel, Meadowsweet, Mullein, Pimpernel, Plantain Leaves, Scouring Rush, Shepherd's Purse, Stinging Nettle, Watercress

ZINC HERBS

Horsetail, Paprika, Shepherd's Purse

HEALING OILS AND TINCTURES

HEALING OIL RECIPE

Take 2 handfuls of fresh herbs or 1 handful of dried herbs. Cover with olive oil. Let stand in a warm place for 14 days, stirring once in a while. After 14 days, simmer for 15 minutes and strain. Squeeze the last drop of oil out of the mixture. Again put 2 handfuls of fresh herbs or 1 handful of dried herbs in the leftover oil and, placing it in a warm place, repeat the procedure. After 14 days, bring it to a boil and simmer it again for 15 minutes. Strain and squeeze out the last drop of oil. There is not much left; however, the oil is mighty potent, and you need only a few drops.

Use the previous recipe for any of the following oils:

CALENDULA OIL

Good for boils and everything that does not want to heal.

CHAMOMILE OIL

Good for cramplike pains.

DILL OIL

Can be rubbed on all aching parts of body.

JUNIPER OIL

Good for cramps in legs, pain in hips, and paralysis.

LILY OIL
Helps spasms, tendons, wrinkles, and scars.

PEPPERMINT OIL
Helps frozen fingers or ears. Good for scars or calluses.

TINCTURE RECIPE
Take any herb, preferably fresh, and place in a jar that has a tight-fitting lid. Cover with 80 proof alcohol (not rubbing alcohol) and let it sit in a warm place for 10 to 14 days, stirring once in a while. After 14 days, strain and pour into bottle. Use small amounts, as it's potent.

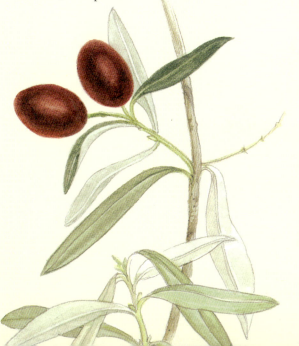

ABOUT THE AUTHOR

HANNA KROEGER is the daughter of German missionaries. She studied nursing at the University of Freiburg, Germany, and worked in a hospital for natural healing under Professor Brauchle. In 1953, she and her family came to America.

After coming to the United States, Hanna took advantage of the education offered by the American systems, ranging from Amerindian herbology to massage. She has a Doctorate of Metaphysics (MsD), and she is an ordained minister in the Universal Church of the Masters, a church well known for its work in contact and spiritual healing. Besides teaching and lecturing, she owns a health food store in Colorado, and has for years owned and operated a health resort, the Peaceful Meadow Retreat, where she has seen her knowledge of nutrition used with exciting results.

For more information on any of the herbs and home remedies in this book, please call Hanna's Herb Shop at: (800) 206-6722.

We hope you enjoyed this Hay House Lifestyles book.
If you would like to receive a free catalog featuring
additional Hay House books and products, or if you
would like information about the Hay Foundation,
please contact:

Hay House, Inc.
P.O. Box 5100
Carlsbad, CA 92018-5100

(760) 431-7695 or (800) 654-5126
(760) 431-6948 (fax) or (800) 650-5115 (fax)

Please visit the Hay House Website at:
www.hayhouse.com